ADRENAL TRANSFORMATION PROTOCOL

ADRENAL TRANSFORMATION PROTOCOL

A 4-Week Plan to Release Stress Symptoms
and Go from Surviving to Thriving

IZABELLA WENTZ, PHARMD, FASCP

AVERY
an imprint of Penguin Random House
New York

AVERY

an imprint of Penguin Random House LLC
penguinrandomhouse.com

Copyright © 2023 by Wentz, LLC
Illustrations by Tina Chan
Images by Dave Kinzel
Cover photography by Ryan Astamendi

Most Avery books are available at special quantity discounts for bulk purchase for sales promotions, premiums, fundraising, and educational needs. Special books or book excerpts also can be created to fit specific needs. For details, write SpecialMarkets @penguinrandomhouse.com.

Library of Congress Cataloging-in-Publication Data

Names: Wentz, Izabella, author.
Title: Adrenal transformation protocol: a 4-week plan to release stress symptoms
    and go from surviving to thriving / Izabella Wentz, PharmD, FASCP.
Description: New York: Avery, an imprint of Penguin Random House LLC, [2023] |
    Includes index.
Identifiers: LCCN 2022033648 (print) | LCCN 2022033649 (ebook) |
    ISBN 9780593420775 (hardcover) | ISBN 9780593420782 (epub)
Subjects: LCSH: Stress (Physiology)—Endocrine aspects. | Adrenal glands—Diseases. |
    Adrenal glands—Diseases—Diet therapy—Recipes.
Classification: LCC RC659.W45 2023 (print) | LCC RC659 (ebook) |
    DDC 616.4/5—dc23/eng/20221202

Printed in the United States of America
1st Printing

Book design by Silverglass Studio

To my dear health-seeking readers who are struggling in this moment—may you recover your health so that you can feel like the calm, beautiful, powerful, and brilliant person you truly are!

Contents

Your Symptoms Are Real—and Reversible

What were you doing in your life before you got sick? This is a question I like to ask my functional medicine clients to help them determine the root cause of their current symptoms and to help develop an effective plan. Functional medicine is a patient-centered approach to healing focused on addressing the root causes of disease, not just the symptoms.

For many of them, the answer is "I was going through a tremendous amount of stress."

Whether it's the stress of everyday modern life, the positive stress that is celebrated, like going to graduate school, starting a new business, or having a brand-new delicious baby, or the type of stress that is grieved, like divorce, a death in the family, or being a victim of a crime, stress can stay with us and cause (or exacerbate) illness.

They say that what doesn't kill you makes you stronger, but based on what I have seen with my clients, a more accurate statement for many of us may be "What doesn't kill you can stay in your body and overwhelm your stress response," leading to a whole host of chronic stress symptoms that weigh us down.

If you're reading this book, there's a good chance that you are not feeling like the best version of you. Perhaps you struggle with fatigue or unrefreshing sleep. Maybe you have trouble remembering everyday things and live in a sea of "brain fog." Perhaps you find yourself more moody than you would like to be, or you become easily overwhelmed with day-to-day life. You may struggle with your weight, insomnia, hormonal imbalances, chronic pain, and perhaps even your libido.

Yet if you're anything like me, or the thousands of people I have supported over the last decade, conventional medicine has offered you very little hope. You may have heard that these symptoms are "normal" or "just in your head," but let me clarify: They are not "normal." They are *common*. Just because they are common, it does not mean that they are normal or that you are stuck with them. I also want to assure you that you are not crazy, the symptoms are not just "in your head," and you've come to the right place. I'm here to take your hand and help you out of the sea of overwhelm to help you shed all that isn't you so that you can shine your brilliant light.

The constellation of frustrating symptoms I have just described that includes feeling tired during the day but "tired and wired" at night, anxiety, insomnia, unrefreshing sleep, mood swings, poor memory, decreased sex drive, cravings for sweets, pain, brain fog, burnout, overwhelm, and exhaustion are typical of a syndrome that is very well known to alternative medicine practitioners and commonly known as adrenal fatigue. According to alternative medicine theories, these symptoms develop as a result of chronic stress, and the answer lies in supporting the adrenal glands, which are small hormone-producing glands that live on top of our kidneys and release our stress hormones.

I turned to the world of alternative medicine and adrenal fatigue in 2009. I was a young pharmacist who had struggled for almost a decade with many frustrating symptoms that were not resolved with conventional treatments. When my integrative doctor first suggested that I get tested for adrenal fatigue, I googled the term and found a "reputable source" that said adrenal fatigue was a made-up disorder and did not exist.

Being a skeptical pharmacist who was taught that "natural remedies did not work," I put off testing my adrenals. I had just ventured into the world of alternative medicine and was always afraid of people trying to take advantage of me and take my money, not realizing that while there are always ill-intentioned people in this world, for the most part, the practitioners I was seeing were simply trying to help.

I brushed off their advice thinking that I knew better. After all, I had a doctorate in pharmacy and was taught that alternative medicine did not work. Yet, despite all of my years studying health, I was walking around exhausted, irritable, and easily startled, with frequent panic attacks, and even showed signs of premature ovarian failure in my twenties. I would have crazy blood sugar swings that left me feeling faint and light-headed, as well as blood pressure that was so low my doctor often wondered how I was able to walk around.

Eventually, I got to the point where I became desperate, and despite my previously tightly held convictions, boy, was I in for a huge surprise. Upon testing my adrenals with an adrenal saliva test, I learned that I did indeed have adrenal fatigue, and lo and behold, the recommended treatments helped me feel so much better in a short amount of time. My anxiety virtually disappeared, and I have not had a panic attack in over a decade. My other symptoms of fatigue, irritability, brain fog, and low blood pressure continued to improve until they were a distant memory.

We now know that the term "adrenal fatigue" is not a physiologically accurate way to describe the cause behind this common symptom cluster; more precise terms are "hypothalamic-pituitary-adrenal axis (HPA axis) dysfunction" or (my preference) "impaired stress response." But the constellation of symptoms does exist, and there are solid treatments that can help. I'll get into the details of the causes of adrenal dysfunction and controversies over correct terminology in later chapters, but for simplicity's sake, I will be using the widely accepted term "adrenal dysfunction" to describe this group of symptoms.

Through my own healing journey and through supporting others on theirs, I have found that with strategic interventions we can significantly reduce or even completely resolve many of those frustrating symptoms while building strength and resilience in the body. I've also found that while lifestyle habits emphasized by integrative medicine practitioners indeed do help, there's often deeper work that needs to be done to truly restore the stress response, and that many of the recommendations, while helpful under the right circumstances, may not work for everyone.

As you are reading this, I want you to know that the symptoms you are experiencing are 100 percent real *and* 100 percent reversible, but I will need you to keep an open mind and an open heart, and truly invest in your healing (because you are worth it!). The program in this book, based on one that has helped thousands of participants dramatically improve their health, is designed to make it easy for you to get at the root cause of your symptoms and address your healing from every angle, sharing with you a few simple lifestyle changes to help you feel happier, calmer, and more energetic, clear-headed, and alive each day.

With every change, your symptoms are going to start transforming. Every day in every way, you will start to feel better and better, and once you are free of those symptoms that sometimes feel like chains that drag you down, you will be able to climb out of the overwhelm. Underneath it all, you will find the beautiful, calm, energetic, and sharp person that you really are.

I'm so glad that you are here and I am so excited to provide you with this tried and tested guidance on how to take charge of your health so that you can thrive.

Do You Have Adrenal Dysfunction?

We will do a full inventory of your symptoms in Chapter 3, but for now, go through this list to see if any of these resonate. Symptoms of poor adrenal function may include the following:

- Feeling overwhelmed
- Feeling tired despite adequate sleep
- Trouble falling asleep or trouble staying asleep
- Difficulty getting up in the morning
- Dependency on caffeine
- Cravings for salty foods (a.k.a. the "I just ate a whole bag of chips" syndrome)
- Cravings for sweet foods
- Increased effort required for everyday activities
- Intolerance to exercise
- Low blood pressure
- Feeling faint/dizzy when getting up quickly
- Easily startled
- Mental fog or trouble concentrating

- Alternating diarrhea/constipation
- Low blood sugar (often presenting as feeling angry when hungry or, as I like to call it, "hangry")
- Decreased sex drive
- Decreased ability to handle stress
- Longer healing time
- Mild depression
- Less enjoyment in life
- Feeling worse after skipping meals
- Increased premenstrual syndrome (PMS)
- Reduced ability to make decisions
- Reduced productivity
- Poor memory

Do any of these sound familiar?

If you have three or more of these symptoms, and if these symptoms developed after experiencing a period of acute or chronic stress, sleep deprivation, an infection, or toxic exposure, chances are that you have adrenal dysfunction. Adrenal dysfunction generally occurs when your HPA axis is unable to effectively manage your stress response. The HPA axis describes the interactive feedback loop that takes place among these three endocrine, or hormone-producing, glands. If the communication among these three breaks down, your adrenals and their ability to produce important essential hormones can be jeopardized.

I know all of these symptoms may seem overwhelming and like a lot to get a handle on. The good news is that turning these around does not have to be complicated. When you start supporting the adrenals—making a few small dietary changes, taking the right supplements—you can produce profound improvements in your symptoms. Just ask some of the participants of the Adrenal Transformation Program, the group program I designed in 2019 and the basis for the Adrenal Transformation Protocol in this book (or the ATP, as we like to call it)!

After completing the program, Angie G. reported feeling "so powerful now, I'm ready to take on the day. I wake less tired. I have joy. I have hope. I am excited to get things done. My anxiety is all but gone now. I am not overwhelmed by my day-to-day, and I'm able to complete tasks without it taking me forever. I want to do more things in life and hang out with people again!"

Constance B. also felt reenergized, sharing, "I'm not tired. I feel mentally clearer. I seem to have more resilience to stress and I feel a lot calmer . . . I generally feel more excited about life."

Anastasia V. felt better than she has in over a decade with "more energy to approach my day. Many of my body aches have diminished. I'm getting quality sleep every night for the whole night!"

Can Your Symptoms Be Resolved?

Through years of research, patient study, and work with thousands of clients, I've found adrenal transformation to be essential for optimal health. While the origins of chronic stress symptoms are many, the body has a very predictable way of breaking down, and I have found that there's a very predictable way of building the body back up in order to thrive.

Regardless of the cause of the stress, the body will respond the same way. In extreme cases, we may need to do some deeper digging to figure out the origins of the stress, but in the meantime, I want to share a predictable method of how to lower your body's stress burden. The chronic stress symptoms you are experiencing are a clue that the major body systems that keep us healthy and thriving—the adrenals, gut, and liver—are compromised. These are the three systems that may require balancing in order to restore the body's natural equilibrium. Because the body is a system, and because the adrenals impact many functions throughout the body, including the body's ability to shift its resources to focus on maintenance and healing, supporting the adrenals is one of the first things I recommend. In approximately 80 percent of cases, addressing the adrenals will result in complete resolution of chronic stress symptoms, and the other two systems self-balancing. In the remaining 20 percent of cases, individual root causes, the gut, and/or liver may also need to be addressed to achieve symptom relief.

My approach to transforming the adrenals has evolved over time, moving beyond old-school alternative adrenal protocols to create a program that I've found to be more comprehensive and effective, yet at the same time more approachable and sustainable for the majority of people. The ATP is designed to calm the nervous system and nourish and rebalance the adrenals, helping to reduce or eliminate many frustrating symptoms and transform our bodies from surviving to thriving. Within weeks, sometimes days, of starting the diet and supplements, you should see some really big improvements, including:

- Fewer blood sugar crashes and less feeling "hangry" (hungry + angry).
- Feeling more in control of your emotions.
- Reduced anxiety, a sense of calmness, and fewer worries.
- An easier time falling asleep and getting quality sleep so that you can wake up feeling more refreshed.
- More joy and happiness!
- An increased ability to handle and cope with stress.
- A healthy and stable blood pressure.
- Improved hormone balance.
- Clearer, sharper thinking . . . goodbye, brain fog!
- Lots of energy!
- The people in your life magically become less annoying (well, not really, but it sure feels like it when your adrenals are balanced).

Over the course of the program, you should notice more symptoms vanishing.

In addition, the ATP will start shifting your body into recovery mode, helping to balance your stress response and gradually building up your strength and resilience to help prevent excess stress from overwhelming your adrenals in the future. You'll know your unique adrenal triggers—and how to avoid them—and have a much stronger foundation to be able to withstand stress when it (inevitably) strikes.

It may feel like stress is a constant in our lives, and that there's nothing we can do to change things or make them better, but with the proper care and support, we can still thrive, even in our modern world. When we are running on empty, every day is difficult, and we feel like we carry the weight of the world on our shoulders. But know that there is a way out, and I am honored to be your guide on this journey. While it may be scary to start down a new path of healing, it is absolutely worth it, and I am here to provide hope and encouragement every step of the way.

I do what I do because I want to help as many people as possible transform their health and their understanding of what's possible for their lives. I want everything and anything to be possible for you. I want you to pursue your passions and achieve your dreams. I want you to have a cup that's so full, you can give from your overflow. I want life to feel like a joy and not a burden to you. I want you to do what fuels you and adds happiness to your life. I want you to know—and believe wholeheartedly—that you are powerful and true healing is possible.

By picking up this book you've taken the first step toward achieving your health goals and shedding the stress symptoms that prevent you from being the you that you are meant to be. Turn the page, and let's take the next step together!

HOW TO USE THIS BOOK

For those of you who want to understand the *why* behind the *what*, Part I explains the science behind the ATP as well as provides inspiring stories and practical strategies for getting the most out of the protocol. If you're the kind of person who just wants to get started already, feel free to turn to Part II for the protocol. But for the very best outcomes, I encourage you not to skip Part I and gain a better understanding of what's going on in your body and how best to support it on your healing journey.

PART I

Understanding Your Adrenals and How Best to Support Them

My Adrenal Success Story—How Thousands Have Healed and You Can Too

When people see me today, they tell me that they just don't believe that I was ever sick, and to be honest, most people never knew that underneath my smiles, I was suffering from numerous mysterious symptoms. The symptoms started during my first year in college and continued to get worse with each passing year. For over a decade, I endured a series of chronic symptoms: debilitating fatigue, irritable bowel syndrome (IBS), anxiety, panic attacks, palpitations, acid reflux, chronic cough, hair loss, dry and dull skin, weight gain, cold intolerance, allergies, carpal tunnel in both arms, brain fog, emotional dysregulation, and muscle and joint pain. Of course I sought the help of numerous doctors . . . but the answers I got were always the same:

> "You're just getting older." I was in my twenties when I heard
> this gem.
> "Maybe you need antidepressants." But I'm not depressed. I just
> have these weird panic attacks that come out of nowhere.
> "Your lab tests are normal." But they didn't do the right ones, and
> at the time, I didn't know any better.

Finally in 2009, after finding a doctor who was willing to do more comprehensive lab testing for me, I was diagnosed with Hashimoto's thyroiditis. Hashimoto's is an autoimmune condition in which the immune system recognizes the thyroid gland as a foreign invader, eventually leading to enough thyroid damage that the thyroid is unable to function properly and cannot produce enough thyroid hormones.

Thyroid hormones regulate metabolism, heart rate, digestion, blood pressure, the menstrual cycle, and body temperature, among other important roles. Every single cell in our bodies depends on thyroid hormones in some way, so when our thyroids are out of balance, we feel it everywhere.

As a pharmacist, I knew a thing or two about the thyroid, but in full disclosure, I thought hypothyroidism was a super-boring condition, with just one drug to treat it (levothyroxine). If you had told me that I would one day become the "Thyroid Pharmacist," I would have surely laughed! But of course, the universe had its own plan. After my own diagnosis, I was dissatisfied that the only recommendation from my well-meaning conventional doctors was to take synthetic thyroid hormone replacement pills. Of course, *as a pharmacist*, I fully support using medication when needed to improve outcomes, but I was also taught the value of lifestyle interventions in pharmacy school.

I was excited to start on thyroid medications, and while the meds did help, I still did not feel 100 percent well. I wanted to do everything in my power to feel like myself again, so my next step was clear: to find a set of lifestyle interventions that would get me 100 percent better.

I reviewed the latest scientific research, online patient forums, and various health books. I consulted with numerous medical experts across a range of disciplines and healing modalities. I turned myself into a human guinea pig and tracked the outcomes of various interventions. After a lot of trial and error, I was able to remarkably improve my health and get my condition into remission through addressing the many imbalances that are present in Hashimoto's, beyond a deficiency in thyroid hormones. They include food sensitivities, blood sugar imbalances, infections, intestinal permeability, nutrient deficiencies, an impaired ability to handle toxins, and, last but not least, an impaired stress response, also known as adrenal dysfunction. I know that addressing these issues can produce profound healing, and it has been my goal to distill the information from emerging research, the insights of functional medicine theory and testing, and my personal and client experiences into accessible self-help guides for self-healers like yourself.

Today, I am able to help others heal because I have healed myself. But to get there, I had to shed a bit of ego and skepticism that initially delayed my own healing.

When my integrative doctor suggested I get tested for adrenal fatigue, I was skeptical. Like most conventionally trained healthcare professionals, I was only familiar with one type of adrenal issue, known as Addison's disease, an autoimmune condition that is life-threatening and requires lifelong use of medications for survival.

When I searched "Dr. Google," I found that "adrenal fatigue" was considered a bogus, "quack" diagnosis. I thought that I knew better, and didn't want to be tricked, so I delayed testing my own adrenals for a long time. It wasn't until I spoke with another pharmacist, Carter Black, RPh (who would later become a wonderful friend and collaborator), about my lingering symptoms and he suggested adrenal testing that I decided to give it a try. Maybe I was more open to it because we had similar training and he wasn't trying to sell me anything, or maybe the timing was just right. I like to think that it was destiny. Sure enough, the integrative adrenal test showed that I had an advanced stage of adrenal dysfunction. I followed the recommended protocols and saw incredible improvements in my energy levels, emotional state, blood sugar issues, and hormone balance—quickly! A lightbulb went off in my head: This works and actually helps!

The Functional Medicine Approach

I wanted to know more about the "how and why" behind these strategies, so I dug deeper into the physiology of the body's stress response and read every book and took every course I could find on the topic. I enrolled in a six-month mentorship training program with Dr. Dan Kalish, a leading voice in stress response protocols, and studied the writings of Dr. James L. Wilson, who coined the term "adrenal fatigue"; Dr. Thomas Guilliams, an expert on stress and the HPA axis and the author of *The Role of Stress and the HPA Axis in Chronic Disease Management*; and the late William G. Timmins, ND, founder of BioHealth Diagnostic and author of *The Chronic Stress Crisis*.

According to Dr. Timmins, the chronic stress response is the body's way of adapting to any kind of stress. In the early phases of chronic stress, the brain and hormonal system pump out large amounts of cortisol. However, as time goes on, the brain and hormone-making organs begin to down-regulate (or minimize) cortisol production to self-preserve, and this leads to low levels of circulating cortisol. I like to call it the "Boy Who Cried Wolf Syndrome." The adrenals were serving up an emergency response to stress but eventually became desensitized to it so that cortisol production remains low.

I learned how the adrenals interact with the hypothalamus and pituitary gland in what's referred to as the hypothalamic-pituitary-adrenal axis, or HPA axis. A communication breakdown among these three, often due to chronic stress, can impair the body's ability to respond to stress in a healthy way and unbalance several hormones produced in the adrenals, such as cortisol, progesterone, and estrogen. This is what can lead to the symptoms I was experiencing, not the adrenals actually being tired.

The more I researched and studied, the more I appreciated the functional medicine approach to adrenal support, based heavily on specific lifestyle changes such as cutting out caffeine, eating for blood sugar balance, and getting lots of sleep (ten to twelve hours!).

The approach also utilizes targeted supplements, most notably the ABCs of adrenal support: adaptogens (herbs that raise the body's resilience to various types of stress), B vitamins, and vitamin C. Additionally, supplements can be used to modify the levels of dehydroepiandrosterone (DHEA) and cortisol, the two most important adrenal hormones. Levels are modified directly through hormone supplements like DHEA and pregnenolone, and/or hydrocortisone, and/or indirectly with magnesium to boost DHEA, licorice to increase cortisol, and/or phosphatidylserine to decrease cortisol.

This approach has worked really, really well for me and for many of my clients with Hashimoto's. As a pharmacist who is passionate about helping others heal, I felt that I really needed to get this healing information to more people, so I shared guidance on adrenal protocols based on these fundamentals in my books *Hashimoto's Thyroiditis: Lifestyle Interventions for Finding and Treating the Root Cause* (2013) and *Hashimoto's Protocol: A 90-Day Plan for Reversing Thyroid Symptoms and Getting Your Life Back* (2017). I have been so humbled by how my own healing journey turned into thousands of healing stories from people around the world who have been able to take charge of their health by using the guides I have written.

In my books, I focused heavily on lifestyle and supplements, as I was limited in my ability to offer specific advice about DHEA, pregnenolone, and hydrocortisone hormone supplementation. During my training I learned that these hormones can have many contraindications and proper use and dosing requires testing; therefore, hormone therapy should only be undertaken with the guidance of a trained professional. Fortunately, the lifestyle and self-care strategies I was able to share still got great results under the right circumstances.

Since developing my initial protocols, I've grown tremendously as a healer. I love to learn from everything and everyone. I am always finding new research, working with clients with unique challenges, taking courses, trying out new interventions on myself, and thinking about how to get more people to feel their absolute best. Equally important, I became a mother and I have to say that my son truly has been my greatest teacher. Since becoming a mom, I have been humbled by motherhood, moms all over the world, and the resilient human spirit. I have learned a great deal about surviving and thriving and the power of oxytocin (the "love hormone") and life's simple pleasures in healing. I've also realized that while some people can undertake intensive lifestyle changes, others need additional healing modalities and gentle options to heal.

As a result, my approach to the adrenals has evolved, just as I have. What I've realized over time is that under the right circumstances the original functional medicine protocols work really, really well but that these interventions are not always possible, feasible, or safe for everyone, every time. So I developed additional protocols that utilized different pathways to produce healing results (and was so excited when I realized that the new protocols often worked even better).

MY ORIGINAL ADRENAL RECOMMENDATIONS IN *HASHIMOTO'S PROTOCOL*

When I originally created the Adrenal Recovery Protocol, these were the main pillars:

- **Rest:** Committing to ten to twelve hours of sleep each night for at least two weeks and kicking caffeine to promote restorative sleep.

- **De-stress:** Using stress-reducing techniques such as gentle exercise and thinking positive to shift the body into a state of relaxing.
- **Reduce inflammation:** Following the Root Cause Paleo Diet to lower the intake of inflammatory foods and increase the intake of anti-inflammatory food.
- **Balance the blood sugar:** Limiting carbohydrates and focusing on eating fats, proteins, and veggies to maintain stable blood sugar.
- **Replenish nutrients and add adaptogens:** Adding adaptogenic herbs, B-complex vitamins, and vitamin C (the ABCs of adrenal balancing) as well as selenium and magnesium.

This approach can provide excellent results under the right circumstances, but, as I've grown as a healer, I've realized that there are additional healing modalities better suited for the real-world challenges of modern life that can provide even better outcomes for more people. The *Adrenal Transformation Protocol* incorporates everything I've learned since developing my initial adrenal recommendations to help you heal and thrive.

A WORD ABOUT SUPPORTING THE ADRENALS WITH HORMONES

I don't recommend supplementing with the hormones hydrocortisone, pregnenolone, and DHEA to balance cortisol production unless you are under the supervision of a knowledgeable practitioner. While these hormones can be helpful when used correctly by the right person, it's important to note that these hormones are potent medicines and need to be tailored to an individual's health history, test results, and genetic profile.

- Hydrocortisone can lead to pituitary suppression when used at the wrong dose or at the wrong time.

- Pregnenolone is the precursor to many other adrenal hormones and has the potential to throw them all off as well as cause fluid retention and extremity pain.
- DHEA can convert into testosterone and estrogen, disrupting the balance of those two hormones, and can over-convert to other, less desirable hormones such as androsterone.
- Testosterone and/or estrogen imbalance can lead to irritability, cystic acne, irregular periods, mood swings, and fatigue, among many other symptoms.
- People who have had or have a risk of estrogen-receptive positive cancers (cancers that bind to estrogen and may need it to grow), estrogen-fueled tumors, or estrogen sensitivities should avoid DHEA due to its potential to turn into estrogen.
- Excess androsterone can lead to symptoms such as acne, hair loss, mood swings, and those lovely chin hairs I have personally experienced.

Rather than give you these external hormones and risk overshooting, we will utilize gentle lifestyle methods that can bring them back to your own unique balance.

When My Original Protocols Worked
for Me and When They Didn't

It was 2017 and four years after I initially healed my adrenals and went on to publish two books on how others could do the same, and I'd burned myself out . . . again. My workload as a health consultant, author, and entrepreneur had drastically increased. I had recently released a documentary series, *The Thyroid Secret*, and published my second book, *Hashimoto's Protocol*. If that wasn't enough, I was writing articles for my website as well as writing for other platforms, engaging with people on all forms of social media, and speaking on radio shows, podcasts, and a variety of media, while trying to manage a team of sixty-plus contractors. I was traveling more often, which contributed to near-constant jet lag and made it tough to stick to my yoga and other stress-relieving routines. I was all-around burning the candle on both ends. One afternoon, when my mom called to say hello and I became annoyed at such an "unreasonable" demand, I knew I'd slipped into full-on adrenal dysfunction and needed to give my adrenals attention. So I did what I was trained to do.

I cut out the caffeine, slept for twelve hours each night, and supported my adrenals with the ABC protocol. I took a sabbatical and de-committed from most of my travel, speaking, and work engagements and focused on relaxing and catching up on things I felt like catching up on. Additionally, my husband, Michael, and I made a plan to scale down and reorganize our business, which allowed for a better work-life balance. And it worked! By following my own proven approach, I saw results in about a month. After that month, I engaged in some advanced protocols I had learned from my colleague Trudy Scott, a nutritionist, mood expert, and author of *The Anti-anxiety Food Solution,* to support the natural production of neurotransmitters due to lingering social anxiety, overwhelm, and lack of motivation that resulted from the nonstop work required to create a nine-part documentary series. (I will share more advanced protocols in Part III.)

After that second bout of burnout, it was an amazing feeling to restore my energy to do my work and continue to help people once more. But nowhere near as amazing as finding out soon after that I was pregnant and my husband and I would be welcoming our first baby.

Pregnancy was a joyful, humbling, scary, and empowering experience all at once. Some days I felt like a plump fertility goddess effortlessly creating a new human being; other days I felt like Humpty Dumpty taking a fall at Home Depot while waiting in the checkout lane. So glamorous, right? ☺

New motherhood was full of wonder, joy, trauma, and shedding of my former self. Everyone knows that having a new baby is a major life change. However, in addition to welcoming my sweet, dreamy bundle of joy, I was faced with additional, less joyful life changes. My super-energetic, marathon-running, early-waking superhero love of my life husband started having some major health issues after a bout of food poisoning, which ultimately resulted in a diagnosis of ulcerative colitis when our son was two weeks old and hemochromatosis (iron overload) a few months later, which required frequent therapeutic blood donations. (Spoiler alert: We were thankfully able to get both conditions into remission, and the focus of my next book will be healing digestive issues, while the hemochromatosis resolved after moving to sea level.) [A quick note on hemochromatosis: Hemochromatosis is usually thought to be a genetic condition, but with my background in functional medicine, I wondered if the environment could play a role. After hours of persistent research and doing lots of tests on my husband, I learned that high-altitude living can lead to an increased production of iron-making red blood cells. Additionally, while my husband's gene reports didn't show the usual hemochromatosis genes, they did show that he had a genetic variation that prevented him from efficiently removing iron from his body. Essentially, he was making more iron but not removing it quickly enough. I came across an obscure foreign research article suggesting that individuals with non-genetic hemochromatosis living at altitude may heal by living at sea level, and after only a year or so of my persuasion, we gave sea-level living a trial, and sure enough, his symptoms began to quickly resolve and his ferritin, a marker of iron overload, was normal within four to six months— which coincides with the 120-day life of a red blood cell! For more guidance on optimizing iron levels, see Iron Toxicity/Overload in the Advanced Stress Symptom Formulary (page 356).]

Beyond worries for my husband's well-being, I felt like my support system vanished. Before the birth of our son, my husband used to jump out of bed and would do a run or hike outside before I woke up, yet after the birth of our son, he was sleeping into the late afternoon and was too exhausted to care for a newborn. I felt torn because I wanted to help my husband heal, yet I needed to mother our son, and I, too, needed to focus on recovering after giving birth (not to mention going back to work and all of the other challenges of new motherhood).

I hadn't found a nanny or even thought about childcare because we had planned that my parents would move to Colorado from Chicago and would care for our son for a few days a week, but unfortunately my parents ended up canceling their move. Instead, my wonderful mom came to stay with us and helped me to care for our son. Knowing that her visit was only temporary (and of course the love for my new baby and my mom), I preferred spending time with both my mom and my son, which prevented me from taking the time I needed to recover.

Our sweet baby boy was delightful (and keeps getting sweeter), and I fell more in love with him every day . . . and like most babies, he woke up every few hours. Sleep deprivation is the number one way to get into adrenal imbalance, and as my sweet boy (and exhaustion) grew, I recognized the signs that my adrenals were getting offtrack again.

Testing confirmed what I'd suspected. And so here I was again, facing adrenal dysfunction, for a third time. But then I hit a major roadblock. Everything about the tried-and-true protocol I'd used in the past seemed impossible at this moment of my life.

No caffeine: ha ha, that just wasn't going to happen. I needed it to get through my day. I'd gotten off caffeine in the past but there was just no way, no how right now. Even though I knew caffeine weakened my adrenals in the long term, caffeine needed to remain a part of my daily routine. I think most new parents can relate. ☺

Sleeping for ten to twelve hours each night for two to four weeks: The idea of getting more sleep was hugely appealing, but not exactly practical. My son needed care and feeding throughout the night. The times my husband tried to help with nighttime caregiving, he would have ulcerative colitis flare-ups from the sleep deprivation. ☹ When I was pregnant, I read a book that suggested children could be night weaned by twelve weeks of age, but due to my son's slow weight gain and feeding challenges, lactation consultants and sleep consultants recommended keeping the night feeds. It would be impossible for me to sleep for six hours, let alone twelve hours straight. Again, it worked great for me before kids, not so much with a little one at home.

Supplemental adrenal hormones, including DHEA and pregnenolone, can work well for some when used in the right doses, under the guidance of a well-trained practitioner, but I wasn't comfortable taking them, as I was still breastfeeding.

I wondered . . . What was I to do? And if this protocol seemed impossible to me, how many other people faced the same challenges? I have always done my best to guide people back to health, and as I was reflecting on my own dilemma, I thought of a few clients who I had not been able to help, despite their best efforts and mine.

I recall a lovely woman by the name of Sheila who was a self-admitted "coffee addict" and woke up frequently at night, struggling with insomnia, anxiety, and pain. She had tried so many things to get better, yet nothing seemed to help. Even when she had quit caffeine, her insomnia and anxiety remained, while her fatigue worsened. Thanks to her, I came to realize that most of us are not sick because we are anxious, caffeine-addicted, and sleep-deprived. Rather, anxiety, caffeine dependence, and insomnia are the consequences and adaptations we develop as part of the stress response.

My passion has always been to help as many people as possible, and it suddenly became clear to me that the original adrenal protocols I'd developed, while effective under the right circumstances, just weren't possible for everyone.

I knew there had to be another way, so I set out to find it so I could help myself and others. I dug in and learned about additional causes and healing modalities through continuing research and education, insights from brilliant and generous colleagues, and of course my own experience and my clients' experiences. This is how the ATP was born. I was the first success story. Despite my sleep deprivation, caffeine dependence, and the many stressors in my life, I was able to not just survive but also heal and then thrive, and today, my little family is thriving as well.

DOES ADRENAL DYSFUNCTION ONLY IMPACT THOSE WITH THYROID ISSUES?

While I came to the world of adrenal fatigue by way of thyroid health, and most people with thyroid issues have adrenal issues, you don't have to have a thyroid or autoimmune condition to have adrenal dysfunction. Adrenal issues may often co-occur with other autoimmune conditions, and periods of extreme stress are a recognized risk factor for numerous chronic and autoimmune conditions.

If you are experiencing the range of puzzling symptoms associated with overburdened adrenals, from anxiety and poor sleep to brain fog, pain, low libido, and fatigue, you will likely benefit from the adrenal program outlined in this book. My hope with this book is to increase awareness about the role the often overlooked adrenals can play in these symptoms and provide help and support to as many people as possible. If you know someone who is struggling with the symptoms of adrenal dysfunction, I hope you'll share this book with them!

The Adrenal Transformation Pilot Program and Results to Date

After I found a way to heal myself for the third time (third time's a charm, right?), I outlined the process so I could share it with others.

I knew that many of my readers with adrenal symptoms needed help, and they aren't always able to connect with a knowledgeable practitioner, and yet I knew that I had to limit my one-on-one clinical work due to my own personal life challenges. I wanted to continue my life's mission to help people heal, so I utilized the time and energy I had to focus on group programs that could empower lots of people to take charge of their own health.

I learned about designing and implementing group programs back in 2011 in my work as a public health consultant. I worked with clinics on creating effective and sustainable patient-care services, including a unique initiative of providing training to patients on self-management of their own health conditions. My first self-management program was inspired by the Diabetes Self-Management Program, which has been clinically shown to improve health outcomes for people with diabetes. Rather than focus on diabetes, I focused on Hashimoto's, and my Hashimoto's Self-Management Program (HSMP) has taught over seventy-six hundred people with Hashimoto's how to take charge of their own health.

As part of this course, I used to teach people how to order and interpret their own adrenal tests. However, one of my favorite lab companies that offered very reliable adrenal testing went out of business. Thus, access to testing and to practitioners who used reliable adrenal testing (and knew how to interpret the tests) became more limited as well. Additionally, DHEA, pregnenolone, and hydrocortisone, the main treatments for adrenal dysfunction, were not available for use over the counter in many places.

I knew that the program would need to be modified for people who would not be able to use adrenal tests and the standard treatments, so I analyzed the labs and my notes on past clients and designed helpful protocols that could be guided by the patient's symptoms, rather than their lab tests, and developed a program that would be guided entirely by symptoms. My team and I released the program to a small group of 213 people in January 2020 and analyzed the results based on symptoms. We improved the program and rereleased it in June 2020 to a larger group of 867 people, then analyzed the results once again and continued this process for two years before the program was converted into this very book you are reading. I wanted to make sure that the program was helpful, safe, and effective for as many people as possible, so we added new strategies, solutions, and guidance with each release. As of March 1, 2022, the program had been released a total of six times with over 2,600 people having successfully followed it. A total of 349 people filled out both the intake and outtake survey, and I am pleased to share the following improvements they reported:

92 percent reduced their mental fog
89 percent experienced less fatigue
89 percent reduced their forgetfulness
86 percent reduced their anxiety
85 percent felt less irritable
83 percent improved their cold tolerance
82 percent improved their morning fatigue
81 percent experienced less trouble sleeping
81 percent improved their libido
80 percent reduced feelings of nervousness
78 percent reduced feelings of depression
77 percent experienced less emotional lability
76 percent reduced their joint pain

The Safety Theory: The Guiding Principle of My Adrenal Transformation Protocol

Our bodies are constantly receiving messages about our environment and adapting to it. Some signals indicate a threat. These include obvious red flags such as an infection or toxin as well as ones you may not have considered such as inadequate sleep, overexercising, erratic blood sugar levels, poor nutrition, intestinal permeability, and mental and emotional stress (a.k.a. life in the modern world). When the body senses danger, the body will react in a way to try to keep us safe and ensure our best chance for survival.

In the face of threat, the body will downregulate our metabolism and repair activities to conserve precious resources and allow for our fight-or-flight stress response to take over and release extra levels of anti-inflammatory, blood-sugar-liberating cortisol. This response can help our survival when used in response to immediate and short-lived threats but can lead to stress-related symptoms when the perceived threat lingers and we don't feel safe.

Our bodies have evolved (or are brilliantly designed?) to adapt to what's needed and maintain equilibrium. A concept referred to as adaptive physiology suggests that our bodies develop chronic illness as an *adaptation* or in response to our environments. I believe that adrenal, immune, and thyroid issues develop as an adaptive mechanism to protect us in times of perceived danger. These conditions help us survive, but in order to feel our best and thrive, we need to figure out what is setting off the danger signals so we can turn them off and make our bodies understand that they're safe.

The good news is that there are many things you can do to make your body feel safe—what I call sending "safety signals"—and every element of the ATP is designed to help you do just that. Through the foods we eat (and don't eat), the ways we act, and the strategies we employ to rest and boost oxytocin (known as the "love hormone"), we can eliminate perceived threats and promote feelings of safety and calm.

Why the Adrenal Transformation Protocol Is Different yet So Helpful

Rather than focusing on tips for a "perfect," unattainable lifestyle to see results, the ATP focuses on sending safety signals and building our resilience so we can thrive in the modern world. This approach acknowledges the real-world challenges that prevent us from pursuing some sort of "perfect" diet or lifestyle, since pursuing perfection can just create more stress. Here are the fundamental ideas behind this new protocol:

- **No Tests Required.** To make this program as accessible as possible, we'll skip the functional medicine adrenal saliva and urine testing during the four-week program. While these tests can be a helpful guide when it comes to understanding possible treatments, they are not required to resolve symptoms for most people. I know that these tests are not widely accessible to many people, and my goal with the ATP is to share easy-to-implement protocols that do not require testing for you to see benefits.

- **Cutting Caffeine Is Optional, as Is Sleeping for Long Periods.** While there are certainly unquestionable benefits of getting lots of sleep and minimizing caffeine, you do not need to sleep for ten to twelve hours each night, nor do you need to quit caffeine (fellow coffee lovers, you can breathe a sigh of relief!). ☺ I've now realized that sleep deprivation and caffeine addiction are *symptoms* of adrenal dysfunction and not necessarily the root cause. To get at the root causes, we will take a different approach—one that addresses the reasons behind what exactly is preventing us from getting quality sleep and why we are so dependent on caffeine. We will focus on solutions that optimize the circadian rhythm, so you can have a lot of energy during the day, and so that you can rest at night. After a few weeks of the adrenal protocol, you should find yourself less reliant on caffeine. If you feel ready to cut back, you'll have an option to do so, but it's just that, an option.

- **Hormone Supplementation Isn't Necessary.** We won't be using hormones like pregnenolone, DHEA, and hydrocortisone. While hormones like pregnenolone and DHEA are available for purchase without a prescription in many countries, they require one-on-one personalized, professional guidance to be used safely and may not be right for everyone. Instead, we will rebalance these hormones naturally, with the use of complementary healing modalities including nutrition, circadian rhythm balance, self-care strategies, and personal transformation work, as well as targeted root-cause interventions.

- **Targeted, Effective Supplementation.** The supplement protocol for the ATP goes beyond the ABCs to address the underlying imbalances most common in people with adrenal issues and utilizes broad-spectrum, multipurpose supplements to solve the most common causes of adrenal dysfunction (such as blood sugar imbalance, sleep deprivation, inflammation, and mitochondrial stress). While these are not required, in my experience, the best outcomes happen when people use supplements, in addition to the other elements of the program.

- **Focus on Making Your Body Feel Safe.** As I firmly believe that adrenal dysfunction develops as an adaptive mechanism to our not feeling safe in our environment, the ATP will restore balance through replacing danger signaling patterns and daily habits that no longer serve us with new ones that support safety and healing.

- **Tools to Transform Your Mindset.** Last but not least, sustainable adrenal hormone balance often requires deep, resilience-building transformational work. Without it, we risk falling into the same old ways and routines that contributed to our adrenal dysfunction and burning ourselves out again and again—no matter how well we follow a blood-sugar-balancing diet. Shedding my past self, letting go of outdated childhood beliefs, and no longer accepting things that don't work for me have been necessary parts of breaking the vicious cycle of healing and crashing my adrenals. Learning how to make the body stronger physically and mentally, shifting into a more self-compassionate mindset, establishing healthy boundaries, and addressing trauma, among other transformative practices, will rewire the way you respond to stress, allowing you to thrive in our modern world. This is where the "transformation" in the ATP comes in!

After healing my adrenals with my new approach, I felt passionate about sharing all that I'd learned to help and empower others in need of an effective, more accessible way to resolve their adrenal dysfunction.

Using the protocols outlined in this book, you can reduce and even eliminate your symptoms and set yourself on a path of increased strength and resilience for many years to come. My goal is to make implementing these healing strategies as easy as possible, with lots of tried-and-true, real-world tips and techniques, support, and motivation along the way. Like me, you are probably juggling multiple demands for your time and attention.

But the truth is, the program only works if you do it. You can feel better, but that will involve making changes to your lifestyle and daily routine. Only you can put those changes into action.

Over the past few years, the Adrenal Transformation online course has helped thousands take back their health, and now I hope it will help do the same for you:

> "I felt like I did over 10 years ago! I'm 57 and I've had the energy that I had when I was 27!! I've been doing tons of work outside (like trimming bushes and weeding—all things I had not been able to do because my joints would hurt so much) and I feel great! No pain. No loss of energy. No need to sleep the next day to recover! My husband has been telling the kids that he can't keep up with me! It used to be the other way around!"—Natasha B.

> "I loved this course. . . . I followed the protocols and feel significant improvements. The brain fog has lifted! My memory has improved. I have less muscle pain, particularly after exercise. I have more energy and better sleep. I handle stress better. I lost weight. What is most important, I feel great!"—Mariana P.

WELCOME, HASHIMOTO'S READERS

If you've read my previous books or joined my online community, I'm honored you're here and to have your continued trust in my ability to provide you with more specific guidance and protocols to support you on your healing journey.

When symptoms such as fatigue, brain fog, low libido, weight issues, anxiety, and joint pain pop up, the thyroid may be blamed. Many of my clients with Hashimoto's thyroiditis will assume they need to take additional thyroid hormones. People with Hashimoto's may initially report feeling more energetic after starting thyroid hormones, but this is usually followed by feeling worse and worse . . . until they are right back to where they were before they started the thyroid medications. At this point, they will likely go back to their physicians to check blood work, only to be told that their thyroid labs are normal.

What most people don't realize, including most conventional medical practitioners, is that the reason behind the symptoms may in fact be due to dysfunctional adrenal hormone output. The adrenal glands release several hormones that impact a multitude of functions throughout the body, including stress tolerance, inflammation, blood sugar, sex drive, and body fat. Adrenal dysfunction causes a cascade of hormone imbalances, including the dysregulation of cortisol, our main "stress" hormone, which has an intricate feedback loop with the thyroid. In the early stages, high cortisol increases antibody production and inhibits the peripheral conversion of T4, the inactive thyroid hormone, to T3, the active thyroid hormone.

At the same time, cortisol promotes the production of reverse T3 (rT3), an inactive thyroid molecule that is able to bind and block T3 hormone receptor sites, thus prohibiting the necessary reactions from taking place and leading to hypothyroid symptoms, despite adequate amounts of thyroid hormones and "normal" thyroid labs (especially when only thyroid stimulating hormone [TSH] is measured). Cortisol also prevents the release of TSH, halting the production of more thyroid hormones. This inhibition is partially to allow cortisol production to occur without interference, as thyroid hormones aid with the breakdown of cortisol to the inactive cortisone.

If the adrenal dysfunction continues, cortisol levels will eventually decline but symptoms of increased reverse T3 will increase. That's because the body, in an attempt to preserve as much active cortisol as possible, will slow down the thyroid to induce hypothyroidism in order to prevent the breakdown of cortisol.

People with hypothyroidism may receive supplemental thyroid hormones to address this imbalance. However, when only thyroid hormone is given, without adrenal support, the person's low cortisol can be further lowered due to the feedback loop. My clients with unresolved adrenal issues often report initially feeling better on thyroid hormones, then feeling worse after starting them.

Active T3 Molecule

The Reverse T3 Molecule

Note that this molecule has one iodine molecule (I) out of place

However, physicians don't routinely check adrenal function in those with Hashimoto's, and most blood tests will not reveal the patterns associated with the type of adrenal dysfunction that is behind the common but not normal stress symptoms. Furthermore, most conventional medicine doctors don't consider adrenal dysfunction a "real" diagnosis, so they don't run the appropriate tests for it, such as adrenal saliva or urinary stress hormone panels.

Supporting the adrenals is an important part of overcoming Hashimoto's and one of the first things I recommend for all of my clients. As I know access to functional medicine testing can be limited, this program is designed to work based on your symptoms, even without access to functional medicine urine and saliva adrenal tests. After utilizing protocols for adrenal balancing, clients have shared that they finally have more energy, lose weight, feel stronger, feel calmer, feel less emotional, and have noticed their libido return.

The ATP in this book provides a deeper focus on how to heal the adrenals based on all that I've learned, including my expanded research and experience, since I wrote the Adrenal Recovery Protocol included in my book *Hashimoto's Protocol,* published in 2017.

How to Get the Most Out of This Program and Be a Success Story

Over the course of the ATP, I will show you how incorporating lifestyle changes into your daily routine can rebalance your stress response and remove the roadblocks that may be hindering your healing. Get ready to give yourself lots of love and positive energy! I encourage you to embrace behaviors that will help you get the most out of this program and that I've found most often lead to success:

- **Have a positive, can-do attitude:** A hopeful, optimistic outlook makes it easier to adopt new strategies while boosting your self-confidence and resilience. If you've been feeling unwell for a while, it's perfectly natural to feel defeated, and even forgo taking action due to the fear that nothing will work, but please remember that even small, positive changes such as our thoughts can set us on a path to healing.
- **Be willing to take action:** Don't let analysis by paralysis prevent you from trying the diet or other strategies.
- **Trust your body:** Listen and honor the messages your body is sending you and trust them to help guide your actions. This includes resting when you need to rest.
- **Accept the support of a loving partner, friend, family member, or support network:** Lean on those who want the best for you. You do not have to be on this journey alone.
- **Be grateful for small gains and improvements and celebrate little successes:** Every positive change to your health and wellness is worth acknowledging. You've worked hard for it!
- **Believe you're worth it:** You deserve to be well and are worth healing. Allocate the amount of time, effort, and resources you are comfortable with to meet your needs.
- **Keep "living":** Live your life to the fullest. Try not to withdraw from the world or put off your dreams and ambitions until you feel better. If you've been afraid to spread your wings because of your symptoms, don't be afraid anymore! I've found that people who don't stop living just because they have a health condition are the ones who experience faster, deeper, and more profound healing.

- **Surrender your need to control every situation:** Letting go of control-freak tendencies can be hard (I know firsthand!), but they contribute to your stress load and hinder your healing.
- **Be patient and persistent:** A change in your health won't happen overnight or because of any one intervention. This book will guide you through protocols to help you get at the root causes driving adrenal imbalance, but only with persistence and patience will you discover what your unique body needs in order to restore balance.

Above all, be kind and gentle with yourself. Healing is a journey. You don't have to be perfect to get better. Every baby step toward healing is a step in the right direction. You're here and you're already doing important work!

WHY DOESN'T MY DOCTOR BELIEVE IN ADRENAL FATIGUE?

If you've looked online to try to find some answers about why you don't feel like yourself anymore, you've probably come across the term "adrenal fatigue" and grown thoroughly confused by all of the conflicting messages about it.

On the one hand are some professional medical organizations, such as the Endocrine Society, stating that "no scientific proof exists to support adrenal fatigue as a true medical condition," and research published in reputable medical journals declaring that a systematic review of nearly sixty studies "proves that there is no substantiation that 'adrenal fatigue' is an actual medical condition. Therefore, adrenal fatigue is still a myth."

On the other are well-known, respected functional, naturopathic, and integrative medical experts acknowledging its existence, explaining how it develops, and offering ways to treat it. To complicate the matter more, some integrative practitioners have now begun to say that adrenal fatigue is a myth.

It's been really interesting for me to realize that what's going on is, in large part, a disagreement over word choice and the proposed physiology behind the cluster of real and frustrating symptoms. The term "adrenal fatigue" was first used by Dr. James L. Wilson in 1998 to identify below-optimal adrenal function resulting from stress. The thinking was that as the adrenals become overwhelmed by stress and excess cortisol release, they become unable to produce sufficient cortisol and other adrenal hormones.

Wilson's new term was a useful way to describe a cluster of symptoms including fatigue, insomnia, and cravings for salty and sweet foods, among others. It also helped to distinguish the condition from Addison's disease (also known as adrenal insufficiency), a rare, life-threatening disorder, in which the adrenal glands are unable to produce enough cortisol. Addison's is usually caused by autoimmune damage to the adrenals, leading to similar but more extreme symptoms such as extreme fatigue, weight loss, darkening of the skin, low blood pressure, and low blood sugar.

As we've learned more about the body and how it responds to stress, we've realized that the original description of the mechanisms behind adrenal fatigue isn't accurate. Most modern integrative practitioners recognize that the adrenals do not become "fatigued," worn out, sleepy, tired, sluggish, or lazy because of chronic stress.

Instead, the new proposed mechanism is that a communication breakdown between the organs of the HPA axis leads to an imbalance of adrenal hormones. The adrenal glands may be physically healthy and perfectly capable of producing adrenal hormones, but because of the communication breakdown, they may not be receiving the message to make them or may produce them at improper times. The term "HPA axis dysfunction" (or "adrenal dysfunction") is now the term that is used to describe the cluster of stress symptoms, as it more accurately describes what's happening in the body. Additionally, the term "hypocortisolism" is used to describe the lowered production of cortisol. Yet, conventional medicine continues to debate the narrowly defined adrenal fatigue, leading to those stunning oversimplifications that the condition does not exist.

Functional medicine expert Marcelle Pick, NP, explained it best when she said, "I focus on the *fatigue*, which is often the worst symptom of this condition we've come to know as adrenal fatigue. And often, that fatigue *is* caused by dysfunction in the adrenal glands, leading to imbalanced cortisol levels. So in that way, the term makes a lot of sense. Perhaps if we called it 'fatigue due to adrenal dysfunction' there would be less debate over whether or not it exists. Whatever we call it, there are very real symptoms that result from dysfunction in the adrenal glands."

Conventional and functional medical practitioners also approach testing and the interpretation of test results differently.

Conventionally trained doctors utilize blood tests and occasionally imaging of the adrenals to look for certain adrenal gland disorders, such as Addison's disease and Cushing syndrome (excessive production of cortisol from the adrenal glands) and the over- or underproduction of adrenal hormones due to nodules or tumors on the adrenals or pituitary gland, and are not well versed in the more broadly defined adrenal dysfunction. They will not utilize the urine and saliva tests used by functional practitioners, as those are usually not covered by insurance, and many people with stress-related symptoms are often told that all of their lab tests are normal, their symptoms are normal, or—worse—that their symptoms are all in their head.

Conventional Medicine Approach to Testing and Interpreting Adrenal Tests	Root Cause Approach to Testing and Interpreting Adrenal Tests
Blood tests for sodium, potassium, cortisol levels, ACTH stimulation tests, insulin-dependent hypoglycemia, 21-hydroxylase antibodies (adrenal antibodies), and imaging of the adrenals to diagnose Addison's disease.	Symptom assessments and tests for cortisol, DHEA, and other hormones via saliva or urine multiple times per day to understand the body's cortisol-release patterns throughout the day.

Conventional Medicine Approach to Testing and Interpreting Adrenal Tests	Root Cause Approach to Testing and Interpreting Adrenal Tests
If tests reveal Addison's disease, hydrocortisone, prednisone, or methylprednisolone is used to replace cortisol, and fludrocortisone is used to replace aldosterone. The medications are required to survive and are used lifelong.	If test results show dysregulated cortisol patterns/levels, the body's stress response requires some attention. Lifestyle changes and supplements are used for three months to two years to eliminate symptoms and to help us thrive.

It's so important to diagnose Addison's disease properly and offer the lifesaving treatments of the steroids the body is no longer able to make. I became well versed in Addison's disease as my own dog, Boomer, is an Addison's patient and conventional veterinary medicine saved his life, and I know that many lives have been saved thanks to doctors who diagnose Addison's in a timely manner in their patients. While I am so grateful for conventional medicine, I also know it can be a challenge to find a healthcare professional who will listen to you and can test for adrenal dysfunction, unless that person is also trained in integrative, lifestyle, or functional medicine as well. One of the reasons I created the ATP and wrote this book is to empower you with an understanding of why your symptoms are happening, as well as the knowledge you need to take back your own health.

What should you take away from all of this?

- What you are experiencing is real. Your symptoms are real.
- The condition is best described as HPA axis dysfunction, adrenal dysfunction, an impaired stress response, or hypocortisolism (in the advanced stages), rather than the narrowly defined "adrenal fatigue."
- Making lifestyle changes to reduce chronic stress and take care of your adrenals and entire HPA axis will help you feel better. I'll be sharing a variety of solid and cutting-edge approaches throughout the book.

You Can Do This

Starting a new protocol is a great opportunity to start fresh! These next four weeks open up time to let go of the past and dream and plan for the future. It's "you" time, a chance to slow down and focus on you. I have high hopes for you and your transformation!

You're probably tired of being tired, tired of spinning your wheels, and tired of spending a lot of money without feeling much better. I know how that feels because I've been there. Even though I'm a healthcare professional, I struggled for too long with fatigue, irritable bowel syndrome, acid reflux, hair loss, carpal tunnel, and anxiety. I had so many doubts about whether I would ever get better, and I sat on my couch each day after work, too tired to do anything other than zone out in front of my television.

At first, my friends and family members thought I was crazy for trying unconventional things. But I persisted, and used my pharmacist training to break down the triggers of my condition, and I recovered. Finally, after I was free from headaches, joint pain, fatigue, bloating, mood swings, and weight struggles, I was able to step into the life that I was meant to live— and you can, too!

The ATP distills the most helpful, approachable, and actionable advice into a practical pathway for healing so that you can start taking back your health right away and begin feeling more vibrant, refreshed, and confident each day.

Here's a preview of what we'll be focusing on to balance your stress response and heal and nourish your adrenals:

- **Balancing blood sugar:** You will see great improvements as you say goodbye to blood sugar crashes.
- **Reducing inflammation:** Removing inflammatory foods can significantly reduce symptoms (sometimes overnight).
- **Replenishing nutrients:** Delicious foods will nourish and support your body back to health. While supplements are not required, you will see additional symptoms resolve and optimal results by using the right ones.
- **Restoring circadian rhythm balance:** Living in sync with your circadian rhythm will help you get the best rest so your body can start repairing itself.

- **Supporting mitochondria:** Through supporting the mitochondria, we will help the body restore optimal energy production.
- **De-stressing:** You will find ways to reduce mental and emotional stress through self-compassion and create sustainable practices that support an ongoing state of thriving.
- **Building resilience:** You will let go of the things that weigh you down, allowing you to be more flexible, and give you the tools you need to recover faster.

No matter where you are on your health journey, I want you to know that you can do this. It's not going to be easy, but you are worth it. I am excited and proud to be here as your guide and cheerleader as you create your own success story.

Chapter 1 Essentials for Your Journey

- If you are experiencing the range of puzzling symptoms associated with overburdened adrenals, from anxiety and poor sleep to brain fog and food cravings, you will likely benefit from adrenal support. While adrenal issues often co-occur with thyroid and other autoimmune conditions, you do not have to have these specific conditions to have adrenal imbalance.
- The ATP is a new approach. Moving beyond traditional functional medicine protocols that emphasize certain lifestyle "choices," such as eliminating caffeine, and testing, the ATP is an accessible way (no testing or hormones) to take charge of your health, heal, and thrive.
- Adrenal issues develop when our bodies feel unsafe. We can send safety signals to the body through the foods we eat (and don't eat) and the ways we act.
- The ATP is designed to make it easy for you to implement healing changes, but only you can put these changes into action. By having a positive attitude and being willing to take action, among other empowering behaviors, you can create your own success story.
- You can do this!

To view the scientific references cited in this chapter, please visit us online at https://thyroidpharmacist.com/atpbooknotes.

Understanding the Origins of Adrenal Dysfunction

If you have adrenal dysfunction, there's a chance that you don't recognize the person you are today. Jessica, a forty-two-year-old real estate agent with two school-aged children, felt like she had lost the person she used to be. She had put on considerable weight, despite dieting, and had constant joint pain and body aches. She was once a triathlete, yet now she was having a difficult time getting in and out of her car for her daily work appointments. Her memory seemed to be failing her, and she worried about losing income because she couldn't keep up with her roster of demanding clients and nonstop deadlines. Her personal life was also a mess. Her husband of fifteen years, whom she considered her soulmate, complained that her libido was now nonexistent. She found herself short-tempered and yelling at her children most days. She used to cherish every moment with her kids, even choosing to take time off work to pull them out of school for special trips, yet now things were different. After a recent outburst over a trivial issue, Jessica found her eight-year-old daughter sobbing in the bathroom. Despite being exhausted all day, Jessica struggled to fall asleep in the evenings and often resorted to a few glasses of wine to help make her drowsy, only to waken in the middle of the night and be fully awake for hours, before being able to go to sleep again!

After a series of blood tests, her doctor had told her everything came back normal even though she felt worse every day. She wasn't sure what to expect from the ATP but wanted to feel like herself again and was enthusiastic about giving it a try. After following the protocol and sending her body numerous safety signals, she was excited to report significant improvements: "I have more energy to approach my day. My body aches have diminished. I'm getting quality sleep every night for the whole night! I feel better than I've felt in over a decade and I'm not snapping at my kids as much. My husband says I've got my sparkle back!"

Like Jessica, many of my clients have reported feeling more like themselves and like the world was a better place after doing the targeted interventions I recommend to address their impaired stress response. The crazy thing is, people see major improvements in symptoms that had been with them for decades, in just two to four weeks. Why do they make such a difference? Our adrenals and the hormones they produce impact nearly every aspect of our physical and emotional health. When our adrenals are in balance, our energy increases, thinking becomes more clear and focused, people magically become less annoying, stress becomes easier to handle, pain lessens, and good-quality sleep comes more naturally.

In some cases, restoring adrenal function may also be key to restoring sex hormones and libido. We were all cheering for one of our program participants when she said, "As I was hugging my dear hubby before he left, it happened!! Hello, hubby, who wants some loving? Ha-ha. Hey, libido, where have you been?! Small victory."

To understand why rebalancing the adrenals can create such positive outcomes—and how adrenal dysfunction happens in the first place—it helps to know more about the adrenals, their role in the body, and what it takes to get them out of survival mode and into thriving mode.

You do not have to become an expert in biochemistry to heal yourself, but I know that for some people, having a good understanding of the background helps with getting on board with all of the protocols (or maybe that's just me?).

The Adrenal Glands

The adrenal glands, often referred to as our stress glands, are two small triangle-shaped organs. One gland sits on top of each kidney. When we are in balance, they produce just the right amount and the right kinds of important hormones to help us deal with stress. The ability to handle stress is essential to our survival. Each adrenal gland has two separate zones, an inner zone, or medulla, and an outer zone, or cortex, that produce different hormones.

The medulla secretes hormones in response to immediate stress. The two most important ones are epinephrine (commonly known as adrenaline) and norepinephrine, which work together to give the body more energy, increasing the heart rate, blood pressure, and blood sugar levels. It also secretes small amounts of dopamine, to promote focus and attention.

The cortex secretes several important hormones made from cholesterol that are important for daily life functions, including cortisol and DHEA. In healthy individuals, this release follows a predictable, rhythmic, circadian pattern throughout the day. Quantities are highest in the morning to help us "get going" and lowest at night so that we can "wind down."

Let's talk about what these important hormones are and how they are made, so that we can understand how key lifestyle changes can make all of the difference in our ability to produce the right amount of hormones at the right time.

1. **Pregnenolone** is the very first hormone produced from cholesterol by the mitochondria of the adrenal cortex and is known as the "mother hormone" because it is the precursor for other hormones (cortisol, aldosterone, DHEA, estrogen, testosterone, and progesterone). Pregnenolone seems to play an important role in healthy aging and memory. Symptoms of low pregnenolone may include forgetfulness, difficulties sustaining attention, fatigue, pain, low libido, and dry skin.

2. **Cortisol, a glucocorticoid,** is the most important adrenal hormone in terms of helping our body adapt to stress. A powerful anti-inflammatory, cortisol regulates blood sugar, supports metabolism, controls body fat, and protects us from infections. You may have heard that cortisol (like cholesterol) is "bad." This is misleading. While high levels of cortisol are problematic, low levels of cortisol are just as troublesome (if not more so) and can lead to debilitating (and even life-threatening) symptoms. We absolutely need cortisol—*in the right amounts.*

3. **Dehydroepiandrosterone (DHEA),** an androgen, is referred to as the "youth hormone" because of its antiaging properties. Its peak production occurs at age twenty and then declines over time. Lower than normal levels of DHEA have been associated with decreased bone density, muscle loss, heart disease, depression, and joint pain. Since DHEA is required to make sex hormones like estrogen and testosterone, insufficient DHEA has been linked to low libido and fertility issues as well. A 2014 study found that women with Hashimoto's and premature ovarian failure, when the ovaries stop producing normal amounts of estrogen or releasing eggs regularly before age forty, were more likely to have low levels of DHEA.

4. **Aldosterone, the primary mineralocorticoid,** helps regulate blood volume, blood pressure, and electrolyte levels. Electrolytes, which help keep us hydrated, include sodium, potassium, calcium, magnesium, chloride, phosphate, and bicarbonate. When this hormone is out of balance, we often experience cravings for salty foods, such as potato chips, a.k.a. the "I just ate a whole bag of chips" syndrome.

5. **Sex hormones: estrogen, progesterone, and testosterone.** While the ovaries are responsible for most of the production of estrogen and progesterone in women, as well as 25 to 30 percent of the testosterone, the adrenal glands also contribute small amounts of progesterone and estrogen to our overall hormone pool, and up to 75 percent of the testosterone in women.

   a. **Progesterone** prepares the body for conception and pregnancy and regulates the menstrual cycle. It is also a "feel-good hormone" because it promotes feelings of calm.

   b. **Estrogen,** the primary female sex hormone, regulates sexual and reproductive health while playing essential roles in the optimal functioning of nearly every organ in the body. It has a major impact on sex drive and sexual arousal, with low levels linked to vaginal dryness, unstable moods, and poor sleep. Hello, low libido!

   c. **Testosterone** is associated most often with men, but women also require small amounts of it to support healthy bones, energy levels, and desire for sex.

THE HORMONES CREATED FROM CHOLESTEROL IN THE ADRENAL CORTEX

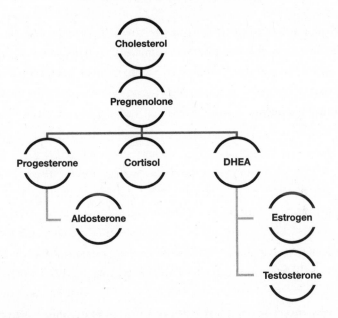

You may have heard that cholesterol is "bad," but cholesterol is actually an important precursor that allows us to make our hormones. Medical professionals know that cholesterol levels increase in pregnancy, when we need to make more estrogen and progesterone; in fact, cholesterol-lowering medications are contraindicated in pregnancy because we would have a shortage of the hormones required for a healthy pregnancy.

However, most people are not aware that excess cholesterol could also be due to the body's response to low hormones, as well as poor conversion of cholesterol into pregnenolone. This is one reason why I don't advocate for low-cholesterol diets; rather, we want to make sure that we have enough cholesterol and that we are optimizing our body to ensure proper conversion into pregnenolone. For proper conversion, we require the healthy function of the mitochondria, which act as gatekeepers for pregnenolone production, and adequate levels of liothyronine (T3, the active thyroid hormone), sunlight, vitamin A (in the retinol form), magnesium, and copper, which act as cofactors for the conversion.

It's important to note that people with hypothyroidism often have high cholesterol and many adrenal symptoms, and it's possibly because of an increased requirement for hormones, coupled with a shortage of cholesterol-converting T3 (and in many cases the other cofactors as well).

If the adrenal glands underproduce or overproduce these hormones, if they don't produce the right amounts of these hormones at the right times, or if the high-cortisol-in-the-morning-to-low-cortisol-in-the-evening rhythm is disturbed, adrenal dysfunction develops. In functional medicine, the primary patterns of adrenal dysfunction are categorized as Stage I (too much cortisol), Stage II (cortisol roller coaster), and Stage III (low cortisol) adrenal dysfunction. In the next chapter, I'll review what happens in each of these stages and show you how you can use your symptoms, including energy levels, blood pressure, hydration status, and how you respond to aerobic exercise, such as running, walking, or biking, to identify your adrenal stage.

For now, let's focus on the causes behind why adrenal dysfunction develops.

What Might Be Preventing the Adrenal Glands from Working as They Should?

There are many reasons why the adrenals may not be able to produce enough cortisol or other adrenal hormones, such as damage to the adrenal or pituitary glands from an immune system attack or a tumor, a genetic disorder, or medications that suppress internal hormone production. In addition, the following causes may contribute to adrenal dysfunction:

- Running out of the raw materials required for proper adrenal hormone production, further contributing to hormone imbalance

- Circadian rhythm disturbances
- The mitochondria are the manufacturing powerhouses where all of the steroid hormones produced by the adrenals are made. Adrenal hormone production can drop off significantly because of impaired or damaged mitochondria.

But most cases of adrenal dysfunction are due to a communication breakdown in the HPA axis caused by chronic stress. It's important to note, the problem is not the adrenal glands themselves. The adrenals are not "so tired that they can't make enough hormones" (as the term "adrenal fatigue" would suggest), but rather that information isn't flowing properly between the glands of the HPA axis.

Getting to Know the HPA Axis

The HPA axis is the intricate feedback loop that takes place between the hormonal control center of our brain (the hypothalamus), the tiny master gland that monitors and manages the hormone excretion of the actual hormone-producing glands (the pituitary), and the adrenal glands that make cortisol.

The hypothalamus is like the CEO of our body's production of hormones. It scans messages from our environment and other hormone-producing glands and checks the body's overall hormonal status before passing on the order for more hormones to the pituitary gland.

The pituitary gland then acts like the project manager, pulling together individual workers (like the thyroid gland and adrenal glands) to do their jobs. The pituitary will also make sure the workers have adequate resources to do their jobs by managing growth and repair, as well as electrolyte/water balance.

When communication is intact among the hypothalamus, pituitary, and a target "worker" organ, such as the adrenals, the flow of hormones runs smoothly. But when communication is disrupted at any point along the way, multiple hormones can become imbalanced. Let's take a look at what happens when the HPA axis works as it should and how the process can unravel.

A Healthy HPA Axis = A Healthy Stress Response

The HPA axis is responsible for helping us handle stress and is designed to deal with cases of acute or immediate threats. An intense in-the-moment perception of threat—being chased by a bear, narrowly avoiding crashing into a car, an argument with your spouse—activates a fight-or-flight response. You may already be familiar with this term, a shorthand for describing two common defense behaviors: becoming aggressive or running away, respectively. It's important to note that two additional responses have been described in stressful psychological situations, including "freeze" (when a person is unable to move, talk, or take action when faced with a threat) and "fawn" (when the person becomes overly agreeable in an attempt to avoid the threat). For our purposes we will use "fight-or-flight" as a general reference to the HPA axis response to stress.

The hypothalamus sets off a hormone cascade to get the body ready to respond to the threat via the sympathetic nervous system. As part of this response, the adrenals pump out extra hormones, and the body goes from the state of relaxing, digesting, and healing, orchestrated by the parasympathetic nervous system, to a survival state. To meet the great, stress-induced demand for epinephrine and cortisol, your body shifts energy and resources away from activities not essential to survival, such as growing beautiful hair, metabolizing nutrients into energy, making hormones, digesting food, repairing itself, and feeling content and relaxed (because why would any of that matter when a bear is chasing you!).

Then, once the threat level has diminished, the demand for emergency levels of hormones settles down, and the body returns to the parasympathetic state, focused on body maintenance and upkeep. This is a healthy and normal stress response that allows the body to bounce back to a thriving state after experiencing acute stress. This is what we want and what we are aiming to restore with this program.

An Impaired HPA Axis = Chronic or Unprocessed Stress

The trouble develops when stress becomes chronic and the fight-or-flight response never turns off. Instead of returning to a parasympathetic healing mode, the body remains stuck in a "high alert" survival state.

Modern stressors such as work deadlines, financial challenges, poor sleep, and processed foods coupled with hidden sources of inflammation ignored by conventional medicine, such as food sensitivities or an imbalanced gut microbiome, have traditionally been enough to keep people in continual stress response and a relentless demand for hormones, especially cortisol, to lower the inflammation. When we add modern life to the series of events that began in 2020, a global pandemic, the loss of loved ones, the loss of jobs and businesses, separation from families, curbed freedoms, racial tensions, and the threat of global war, we have a perfect storm for a chronically overwhelmed stress response.

At first, the demand for cortisol is high and the adrenals kick into overdrive to produce enough. Making more cortisol requires more pregnenolone, the "mother hormone," which is also used to make DHEA and progesterone. As cortisol production ramps up, synthesis of these other hormones declines, likely a protective mechanism intended to help us have enough cortisol to survive the stress. But if this goes on for too long, it can lead to deficiencies in the other hormones that are made from pregnenolone.

The intense and immediate demand for hormones due to chronic stress puts the entire stress response on overdrive, leaving room for a communication breakdown between the players in the HPA axis to occur. Excess cortisol for prolonged periods is damaging to the body and eventually, in an act of self-preservation, the HPA axis adapts or downregulates and stops sending messages to the adrenals to produce cortisol. The adrenals are still capable of producing cortisol and DHEA, but they just don't release as much.

Symptoms over Time

If chronic stress persists and adrenal dysfunction progresses from the beginning high-cortisol stage to the advanced low-cortisol stage, certain symptoms and conditions can occur, including:

- Low blood pressure, which happens in the advanced stages of adrenal dysfunction as aldosterone production becomes depleted and levels of sodium and water drop (you might feel faint upon standing as a result of low blood pressure)
- Noticeable dehydration and cravings for salty foods (hello, potato chips!) and possibly an increase in potassium levels (this can be marginal and still within the normal reference range); you may find foods containing high amounts of potassium might make you feel worse, and that drinking more fluids will only result in further

dilution of sodium and increased dehydration (wherever sodium goes, water follows)

- Menstrual irregularities, infertility, low libido, uterine fibroids, fibrocystic breasts, and a shift in immune function, all as a result of low progesterone
- Elevated levels of cholesterol, due to the body compensating for the increased need for this hormone-building material or due to poor conversion into pregnenolone
- Seasonal depression, post-traumatic stress disorder, hypothyroidism, asthma, eczema, inflammatory bowel disease, rheumatoid arthritis, myalgic encephalomyelitis/chronic fatigue syndrome (ME/CFS), fibromyalgia, and premature ovarian failure, which are linked to abnormally low levels of DHEA and progesterone and HPA axis malfunction

THE CONSEQUENCES OF THE CHRONIC STRESS RESPONSE: THE PARASYMPATHETIC NERVOUS SYSTEM VS. THE SYMPATHETIC NERVOUS SYSTEM

Many functions in our bodies happen without us having to think about them, such as breathing, digesting, and the heartbeat. The autonomic nervous system (to help me remember it better during pharmacy school, I would call it the "automatic" nervous system) controls these systems, and it's divided into two parts that oppose each other like opposite sides of the same coin:

The parasympathetic nervous system: Responsible for the "rest and digest" state when the body is able to relax, conserve energy, repair any damaged tissues, and all in all maintain healthy bodily functions. This is the sweet spot for healing the body and is considered an anabolic state, as the body is building itself up.

The sympathetic nervous system: Excess cortisol activates the fight-or-flight response, triggering the release of chemical messengers that cause physiological changes to prepare the body to respond to a stressful situation: Heart rate increases, breathing quickens, and blood sugar and fats flood the bloodstream to fuel higher energy demands. Immediate survival is the priority and everything else, such as digesting food, making reproductive hormones, or repairing tissues, is shelved. The sympathetic state of the body is considered to be a catabolic state, where the body is breaking itself down. While it may be difficult to know that you are in a sympathetic-dominant state, especially if you've been in it for too long, one sign that you may be currently in a sympathetic state is sensitivity to bright lights because our pupils tend to dilate in the sympathetic state.

When the body spends too much time in the sympathetic nervous system state, it's unable to keep up with maintenance and repair. Think of how your house would look if you threw a party every day (or hosted a daily one-hour playdate with just two toddlers ☺) and never took a break to clean up. It would become quite a mess in a very short amount of time! The body cannot thrive in a constant state of fight-or-flight, but a continuous parasympathetic nervous system state isn't ideal, either. We need both systems running well so that we have all of the resources we need to sprint from a tiger and repair damage and build strength. Balance is the key.

....

THE CAUSE BEHIND THE SYMPTOMS

If the disagreement between conventionally and holistically trained practitioners about "adrenal fatigue" wasn't enough, there's also a disagreement between practitioners about the origins of adrenal dysfunction and what leads to depleted levels of cortisol, sometimes called hypocortisolism.

In conventional medicine, the recognized reasons for low cortisol include an autoimmune attack on the adrenals or complications of the pituitary gland. In functional and holistic medicine, I have seen various experts claim that adrenal dysfunction does not exist, rather that people's symptoms are due to a unique cause they have discovered or that they specialize in. Copper toxicity, lack of sleep, circadian rhythm imbalances (including seasonal affective disorder), mold toxicity, sleep apnea, childhood trauma, post-traumatic stress disorder, nutrient deficiencies including the vitamins A, B (especially pantothenic acid and thiamine), and C; magnesium deficiency; neurotransmitter imbalance; pyroluria (a condition associated with low B_6/zinc levels); mitochondrial dysfunction; and a lack of cortisol precursors due to a low cholesterol diet are some suggested causes.

In my experience, multiple causes can lead to the same symptoms, just as the same one cause can lead to different symptoms. This is because the body has a predictable way in which it responds when it's placed under a significant amount of stress. First, it will make more cortisol, then it will start suppressing cortisol production.

Generally speaking, anything that the body perceives as stress can overwhelm the body and lead it into an impaired stress response. The ATP incorporates various healing modalities and root cause solutions to rebalance the stress response and guide you back to your health, regardless of the cause. Rest assured, we will cover all of our bases. The four-week program will help you cut the low-hanging branches, and if needed, Part III will help you dig at the roots.

The Top Four Types of Chronic Stress Sabotaging Your Adrenals

Getting to know the types of chronic stress making the body feel unsafe and driving an overactive fight-or-flight response is the first step in lowering their impact on us. Keep in mind that "stress" is broadly defined as anything that impacts the body's natural balance (called homeostasis), but it's not a pie-in-the-sky, vague New Age concept, rather a real, measurable, predictable, physiological response to perceived threats causing a burden on the HPA axis.

There are four main categories of stress:

1. Inflammation (chronic or acute)
2. Circadian rhythm imbalances
3. Nutritional imbalances
4. Psychological stress (past and current)

Let's take a closer look at the top four.

Top Stressor #1: Inflammation

Inflammation is the body's response to injury. When cells are damaged for any reason, for example, due to a wound, infection, or toxin, the immune system responds by increasing blood flow to the area and releasing healing chemicals and hormones, such as cortisol, to help repair the injury. This process can cause redness, warmth, and swelling (a.k.a. inflammation). If you've ever twisted an ankle and watched it balloon up painfully, you'll have a good idea of what inflammation looks and feels like. Not all inflammation is visible, though. Inflammation is considered chronic when it persists for a long time because the body is unable to fix the problem area.

The most common sources of chronic inflammation I see are due to pro-inflammatory foods, including foods we are sensitive to, as well as intestinal permeability from an imbalance of bacteria in the gut (gut dysbiosis), small intestinal bacterial overgrowth (SIBO), and gut pathogens including *Helicobacter pylori* (*H. pylori*), *Blastocystis hominis*, and yeast overgrowth/ *Candida*.

Chronic inflammation may also occur from a variety of obvious and not so obvious sources, such as injury, obesity, sleep apnea, environmental toxins (radiation, chemical exposure, air pollution, mold, substance abuse, alcohol, certain medications, copper toxicity, iron overload), viral infections (such as Epstein-Barr virus), and lifestyle choices like overwork, overexercising, and not exercising enough.

The ongoing demand for anti-inflammatory cortisol to neutralize chronic inflammation can throw off the HPA axis and trigger adrenal dysfunction.

THE IMPORTANCE OF GUT HEALTH

What does the gut have to do with adrenal balance? A lot! In the areas of natural and functional medicine, there is a widely held understanding that all disease (and thereby all healing) begins in the gut. And for good reason!

The gut performs the all-important role of digesting and absorbing the nutrients we take in, but it also helps regulate the immune system and plays a profound impact on mental state. Often referred to as the "second brain," the gut is in constant communication with the brain in our heads and produces many of the neurotransmitters associated with mood, such as the "happy" hormone serotonin.

The gut is home to trillions of bacteria and functions best when there is a balanced ratio of probiotic (beneficial) and opportunistic (potentially problematic) bacteria. Imbalanced bacterial flora—when there are more opportunistic than probiotic bacteria—is called gut dysbiosis and can cause stomach pain, digestive distress (diarrhea, constipation, bloating), acid reflux, and food sensitivities. An imbalance of gut bacteria also contributes to another common type of gut dysfunction: intestinal permeability, or leaky gut. Harmful bacteria can release toxins that contribute to the loosening of the junctions between the epithelial cells (cells that line the small intestine). When this happens, toxic substances—partially digested food, pollen, feces, dead cells, and bacteria—escape from the digestive system and pass into the bloodstream, triggering an immune response, widespread inflammation, and the stress response.

While there are numerous factors that can cause gut imbalance, I've found that by replenishing beneficial bacteria and strengthening the gut wall by eliminating reactive foods, addressing nutrient deficiencies, eating gut-supporting foods, and supplementing with probiotics and digestive enzymes, most people will see significant improvement in their gut and adrenal symptoms. You'll learn more about these strategies over the course of the *Adrenal Transformation Protocol*!

Top Stressor #2: Circadian Rhythm Imbalances

I spent much of my life feeling tired even after being in bed for over eleven hours each night. I was actually sleeping too much (a condition called hypersomnia), but the quality of my sleep was poor and lacking sufficient restorative sleep so I'd wake up feeling so drained, it was as if I'd never gone to sleep at all. Poor sleep (both quality and quantity) is a huge stressor on the body and a major contributor to many health problems, including adrenal imbalance, and has been linked to inflammation, impaired blood sugar balance, weight gain, and compromised muscle and tissue repair, among other health risks. In fact, all-cause mortality rates are three times higher in sleep-deprived people! One of the fastest ways to induce adrenal dysfunction is through sleep deprivation. In fact, sleep deprivation is what scientists use to induce HPA axis dysfunction in laboratory animals!

Sleep is the primary healing time for both our bodies and our minds; when we don't get enough, our HPA axis suffers. Most adults require between seven and nine hours of sleep (those with chronic illness may need more), including enough body-restorative "deep" sleep as well as brain-restorative rapid eye movement (REM) sleep to function optimally. "Deep" or slow-wave sleep promotes muscle repair and metabolism and good immune system function while REM sleep allows the brain time to consolidate memories, filtering out the unimportant information it received during the day and moving important information from our short-term memory to our long-term memory.

Many of us don't get enough high-quality sleep because our circadian rhythm, the body's natural twenty-four-hour biological clock, is out of balance. When the circadian rhythm is in balance, cortisol floods the body in the morning to help us feel energetic when the sun is out and gradually declines throughout the day, reaching a low point at night to encourage sleep. When that rhythm is thrown off and the optimal pattern of cortisol is disrupted, we may have trouble waking up, be fatigued during the day, and experience trouble falling and staying asleep. Additionally, we are more vulnerable to infection, increased sugar cravings, digestive issues, and night hunger. Furthermore, circadian rhythm imbalance has been tied to seasonal affective disorder (or, as I like to call it, sunshine and light deficiency).

Lights and screens that make nighttime seem as bright as daytime, too much time spent indoors, a lack of sunlight in the morning, jet lag, and shift work can all throw the rhythm off, negatively impact our sleep, and lead to adrenal dysfunction.

Top Stressor #3: Nutritional Imbalances

What we eat—or don't eat!—can put stress on the body. Nutrient imbalances can be grouped into two main categories: nutrient deficiencies and blood sugar imbalance.

Nutrient Deficiencies

Certain macronutrients and micronutrients are required for proper adrenal function, and without a sufficient supply the adrenals will struggle to keep up with adequate hormone production. Nutrient deficiencies can occur as a result of:

- Eating nutrient-poor foods (including conventionally grown and raised foods, as they have been found to be lower in nutrients than organic options)
- Eating foods with less bioavailable (easily and readily absorbed and used) nutrients
- Following a calorie-restricted diet
- Having inflammation from infections or food sensitivities
- Taking certain medications
- Having an imbalance of gut bacteria
- Having low stomach acid or a lack of digestive enzymes
- Having a lack of sufficient thyroid hormones

These nutrient deficiencies add to the body's stress load, and the stress response depletes these nutrients even more, burning through them at a high rate. If supplies aren't replenished, the body enters a catabolic state, breaking itself down for nutrients to fuel the adrenals and, consequently, ratcheting up the stress level even higher. If we're in this catabolic state for a prolonged period of time, we're likely to experience severe nutrient deficiencies as well as perpetuate and exacerbate our adrenal dysfunction. It's a cycle that can be difficult to break.

The most relevant nutrient deficiencies include:

- Healthy fats
- Protein
- Vitamin A
- B vitamins
- Vitamin C
- Vitamin D
- Iron
- Magnesium
- Sodium

Blood Sugar Imbalance

I wasn't aware that I had blood sugar issues when I was first digging into the root causes of my thyroid and adrenal issues (despite being a self-admitted sugar addict). I was thin—therefore, I assumed that I was healthy. However, I would get "hangry" multiple times per day, as the high-carbohydrate foods I had consumed were causing me to experience huge blood sugar swings. What I didn't know was that these swings were also weakening my adrenals.

Blood sugar, also called glucose, is an important energy source for the body, providing nutrients to the organs, muscles, and nervous system. It is primarily obtained from the carbohydrates found in the foods we eat.

Common Symptoms of Blood Sugar Imbalance

- Hormonal issues
- Fatigue
- Depression
- Anxiety
- Insomnia
- Chronic pain
- Poor cognitive function (brain fog, trouble concentrating)
- Hanger (hunger + anger)
- Nervousness
- Light-headedness

When we eat foods containing carbohydrates, the carbohydrates are broken down into glucose that is then released into the bloodstream through

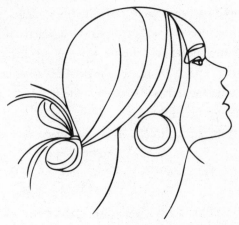

Don't hate me for the things I said when I was "hangry."

the small intestine. Elevated blood sugar signals the pancreas to release insulin. Insulin is a hormone that helps restore balance by shuttling glucose from the bloodstream into cells where it can be used for energy and stimulates the liver to convert excess glucose into glycogen for storage.

Problems arise when we consume large amounts of sugar—and I'm not just talking about desserts—high-carbohydrate foods such as grains and even starchy vegetables are an issue as well—and the pancreas has to release larger amounts of insulin to bring the levels of sugar in the blood back down. These surges in insulin can cause blood sugar levels to drop too low, leading to nervousness, light-headedness, anxiety, low energy levels, and cravings for more carbohydrate-rich foods. Hello, "hanger"! This starts the cycle all over again as blood sugar levels swing high and low. Over time, cells can grow less responsive to insulin so that glucose has a hard time moving into them from the bloodstream. When this happens, known as insulin resistance, the pancreas compensates by pumping out more and more insulin to try to normalize blood sugar levels, amplifying the highs—and lows—of blood sugar swings.

The body prefers to keep blood sugar levels in a normal, steady range, so wild ups and downs put stress on the body, and especially the adrenals, as it tries to restore equilibrium. When the adrenals become stressed, they release an excess of cortisol and our liver gets the message to make more glucose by breaking down muscles for their amino acids (gluconeogenesis), which can lead to hyperglycemia and insulin resistance. In turn, when we don't have enough cortisol, our liver doesn't make enough glucose, and we end up with low blood sugar.

Excess cortisol release also leads to an increased production of inflammatory proteins that are associated with a heightened immune response and autoimmune conditions, such as Hashimoto's, celiac disease, polycystic ovarian syndrome (PCOS), inflammatory bowel disease (IBD), rheumatoid arthritis, and lupus. Blood sugar imbalances have been described as adding "fuel to the fire" of autoimmune disease by many practitioners who focus on reversing these conditions.

Stabilizing blood sugar is an important part of protecting your adrenals from excess stress and healing from autoimmune conditions.

Top Stressor #4: Psychological Stress (Past and Current)
It is likely no surprise that psychological stress may be at the root of an impaired stress response. Feelings such as grief, guilt, fear, anxiety, excitement, and embarrassment can be classified as stress. This stress is based on our perception, not on the nature of the individual stress. For example, large gatherings may cause plenty of mental stress for someone who is an introvert or has social anxiety, while another person who identifies as an extrovert may perceive the experience as pleasurable. Situations that are new, unpredictable, and threaten our sense of self, or that involve feeling a loss of control, are often perceived as stressful, for example, the loss of a loved one, divorce, financial strain, a job change, or any of the alarming world-testing events affecting us daily. But even some of the best moments of our lives can be perceived as stressful, like getting married, going to graduate school, or adding a little bundle of joy to the family.

Mundane, day-to-day things can cause stress, too—a text message from a demanding boss, a constantly cluttered house, an overdue bill, never-ending piles of laundry, or a computer meltdown can throw us into survival mode. And because these "threats" are near-constant most days, we can stay there much longer than we should.

While stress can arise from circumstances outside of our control, it can also be created by beliefs we hold about ourselves and the world. In my case, because of various experiences in my early life, I came to believe the world was not a safe place, that I was not enough, and that I had to take care of myself. This led me to develop trust and control issues, extremely high standards for myself, and perfectionist and workaholic tendencies. In some ways, these coping mechanisms helped me get ahead in life, but over time, as my body started rejecting the all-nighters, the overcommitments, the caffeine, and the busy binges, I kept pushing on and lost my health. Left unaddressed, hardwired thought patterns such as perfectionism can drive our stress response and inhibit our healing, even if we do every other lifestyle change . . . well, perfectly! ☺

An overactive fight-or-flight response is often present in people with a history of trauma. Traumatic events, such as an accident, abuse, or assault, can put us into a sustained fight-or-flight response that makes us keep going, even when our brain and body need to rest, digest, and heal. Childhood trauma has been especially relevant in setting the tone for altered hormone patterns in adulthood. We may not think an experience from our past (even one we don't remember) has the power to influence us, but the body remembers and tries to protect us through the stress response. If the *psychological* trauma remains unresolved and our emotions suppressed, we may find it difficult to heal adrenal dysfunction despite our best efforts with *physiological*-driven lifestyle changes (replenishing nutrients, balancing blood sugar, curbing inflammation). When we are stuck in the fight-or-flight response, our bodies will continue to feel unsafe. Until we restore a sense of safety, both physically and psychologically, there is a high likelihood a chronic pattern of adrenal hormone dysfunction will persist. The good news is that there are many beneficial treatments and therapies to help you recover from your past and take back your health and your life.

I know from my own experience as well as my work with so many clients that addressing psychological stress may be the hardest part of transforming the adrenals. But it is absolutely the most important strategy and I want to assure you: We *can* shift our perceptions of stress and our mindsets to make stress easier to handle and resolve underlying emotional trauma to restore balance to our bodies.

ADVERSE CHILDHOOD EXPERIENCES (ACES)

Emotional abuse, neglect, and household dysfunction experienced in childhood, collectively referred to as adverse childhood experiences, or ACEs, are linked to an increased risk of adult chronic conditions such as Hashimoto's and other autoimmune conditions, heart disease, diabetes, and depression.

How could ACEs exert such a powerful and lasting impact on physical and emotional health? Research suggests ACEs cause a prolonged or excessive activation of the stress response—ultimately, HPA axis dysfunction—which over time can disrupt the development of the immune, nervous, and endocrine systems.

Many people report ACEs, so if you know or think you've experienced this type of trauma, you are not alone.

How to Heal

Now that you have a clear sense of why adrenal issues develop, let's look ahead to a plan for healing using a root cause approach. Through interventions such as balancing blood sugar, replenishing nutrients, re-syncing with the circadian rhythm, releasing inflammation, and self-compassion, we will be sending your body safety signals to dial down its sense of being in perpetual danger. This will then restore the HPA axis communication pathway, transform your adrenals, and reduce or eliminate many of those symptoms!

Chapter 2 Essentials for Your Journey

- A communication breakdown among the hypothalamus, pituitary gland, and adrenals (the HPA axis) is often at the root of adrenal dysfunction.
- Chronic stress can drive the constant activation of the stress, or flight-or-flight, response. This keeps our bodies in survival mode and prevents them from relaxing, digesting, and healing.

- The top four types of chronic stress sabotaging your adrenals and causing your symptoms are inflammation, circadian rhythm imbalances, nutrient imbalances, and psychological stress (past and current).
- The ATP addresses each of those stressors and will help no matter what the cause of adrenal imbalance. Get ready for healing!

To view the scientific references cited in this chapter, please visit us online at https://thyroidpharmacist.com/atpbooknotes.

CHAPTER 3

How the Adrenal Transformation Protocol Can Help You Recover Your Health

The guiding principle of the ATP is to communicate to your body in a language that it understands that it is safe, allowing it and encouraging it to heal. Once your body feels safe, it can move out of survival mode, start thriving, and become more resilient.

To help you feel stronger and more energetic each day, we're going to use a few proven strategies to address the top four chronic stressors sending danger signals to your body and sabotaging your adrenals. For me and the thousands of people I've had the honor of guiding, a holistic approach utilizing various healing modalities focused on restoring healthy HPA axis function has been the most effective strategy for short- and long-term results. Through nourishing and replenishing our bodies with yummy nutrient-dense foods and targeted supplementation, self-care modalities that help us rest and reset (a.k.a. adding more of what makes you feel good!), and gentle resilience-building nudges, the ATP will help move your body from fight-or-flight mode into healing mode.

If the anticipation of making changes or beginning a new program gives you butterflies, I hope sharing some of the remarkable results of clients who have transformed their health and are pursuing their goals and dreams will bring home how powerful small changes can be. Like Heidi P., who has been living with Hashimoto's for twenty-five years and could hardly get off the couch because of exhaustion but today has her energy back.

Or Genevieve, who is now "waking up in the morning and feeling ready for the day instead of wondering if I even slept!"

And Barbara B., who came to appreciate the role of self-care and emotional healing as part of her physical transformation: "I am feeling better. My energy level has improved, my joint pain is much improved and [I've noticed] a reduction in brain fog, headaches, and anxiety. The fact that I am feeling better is an inspiration to want to continue to use the program and to make many of the things we have learned lifelong habits and routines!"

The Adrenal Transformation Protocol

The ATP shows you how to support your adrenals and repair your stress response so you can start feeling calmer, rested, and more alive right away. We're going to transform your energy levels, your symptoms, and your understanding of who you are and what you're capable of. During my evolution as a healer, I have come to learn about so many unique and powerful healing modalities that work together in synergy to help you thrive. Be prepared to see exciting changes to your health and life! Here's how we'll do it:

Replenish

Nutrition, or food pharmacology, as I like to call it, is one of the most powerful ways to send safety signals to our bodies. Remember, feeling unsafe or under threat throws the body into fight-or-flight mode. To feel good, we must send our bodies signals to let them know they're safe and can rest, digest, and heal. Nourishing them with plenty of nutrient-dense foods, eating frequently, and restricting ones that trigger blood sugar imbalance and inflammation is one way to communicate to our bodies that there is an abundance of food and that we are safe. You'll start a diet that nourishes the body while removing the most common inflammatory foods and promoting blood sugar balance. You will discover how to replace reactive foods with plenty of supportive ones—this isn't about cutting or counting calories!—and how this can make a world of difference in healing your adrenals and relieving your symptoms, often in a very short amount of time. Dozens of simple, delicious recipes make following the diet easy. People report major breakthroughs in persistent symptoms after implementing the nourishing, anti-inflammatory, and blood sugar–balancing diet protocols.

Additionally, vitamins, supplements, and herbs, when used strategically, can produce incredible health benefits. Though not required, but highly recommended, incorporating a small number of key supplements can help ease stress, lower inflammation, steady blood sugar levels, and restore depleted nutrients to accelerate your healing. I've chosen six core supplements to help you feel better. Some of them will allow you to experience benefits in as little as two or three days. Others might take a little bit longer to kick in, but you should start feeling stronger and more energized, and notice your symptoms going away overall within weeks.

ATP SUCCESS STORIES

"After starting this program, I feel so powerful. Now, I'm ready to take on the day. I wake less tired. I have joy. I have hope. I am excited to get things done. My anxiety is all but gone now. I am not overwhelmed by my day-to-day, and I'm able to complete tasks without it taking me forever. I'm wanting to do more things in life and hang out with people again! My blood sugar has stabilized and I enjoy the high-protein meals/snacks that help with that. My life has drastically changed for the best and I highly recommend trying this program for yourself if you would like a life change in a short amount of time!"—BETH G.

"I attribute my lessened anxiety to the supplements. They are very professionally, very smartly designed to support the body in the most [gentle] way. Nothing extra, but nothing missing . . . Eliminating my anxiety was due to feeding my body correctly and the supplements controlled the deficiencies that I had."—TATIANA S.

"I think the diet change gave me the most noticeable improvement. . . . This program helped me lose inflammation in my knee from a fall years ago. I lost 7 pounds. After the first week with the diet changes I could tell a difference. With the supplements and diet changes, I feel like the version of me from over 20 years ago if I get enough rest. My body is healing and I have to make rest a priority. I have lost weight and inflammation in my joints. I actually feel better when I get enough rest."—RHONDA C.

Reenergize

Diet changes can give a major boost to energy levels, but there's more we can do to fight fatigue, improve mood, sharpen thinking, and get better sleep. I'll share strategies to ensure proper hydration and electrolyte balance, which are critical for the optimal functioning of every cell. Even mild dehydration means that a system-wide slowdown can result in sleepiness, muscle weakness, fuzzy thinking, and mood swings. We can fix that! You'll also discover how simple lifestyle changes and the timing of certain daily activities can increase energy levels while helping to balance hormones and improve digestion, sleep, and libido by supporting the mitochondria and restoring circadian rhythm balance. You'll see how optimized sleep will allow you to properly heal—and wake up refreshed!

ATP SUCCESS STORIES

"Adjusting my diet and adding the supplements have given my body a new strength! I feel more energized and now sleep deeply and for longer. This means I awake refreshed and able to get out of bed with energy that was previously so elusive to me!"—JANIE G.

"After a few weeks of following these lifestyle interventions, I began to feel more energized and productive throughout the day. My afternoon slump improved, and I had more mental clarity throughout the day."—ZEE M.

Revitalize

We will leverage the healing power of pleasurable activities that make you feel good. You'll send your body safety signals by treating yourself with extra love and compassion. We all know that the actions, thoughts, and emotions that make us feel good help us rest, reset, and recover, but many of us feel like we need permission to do them. Consider this your prescription to do pleasurable activities you enjoy! You'll discover several ways to boost the love hormone oxytocin, such as physical touch, aromatherapy, and sunshine; empower yourself with positive thoughts and affirmations; and feel the healing power of expressing your creativity.

ATP SUCCESS STORIES

"[This program is] life changing. Positive thinking, forgiveness, supplements. So many things helped me overall and then my family felt my change and their personality changed!! I'm so very thankful for this program. You have changed our lives!!!! Much love."—SHERRY

"I have felt more joy, hope, and feelings like I could take on more in the world. It's been exciting to feel so good! My anxiety has pretty much all but gone away. . . . Mindfulness, yoga, and meditation have helped me a lot to reduce tension, exercise, stay strong, and center myself."—BETH G.

"My cravings for salty and sugary food are gone. The ATP is filled with an abundance of ways and means to combat adrenal issues. It not only provides help with choosing healing foods, supplements, and proper exercise, it also offers powerful exercises and support systems designed to uncover, address, and help heal any mental and emotional trauma that contributed to adrenal problems and may interfere with continuing the recovery."—LORI D.

Rebuild Resilience

In this section, we will employ the powerful healing modalities of personal transformation. There are so many effective strategies we can use to increase our body's ability to react to stress with more balance. We'll start by tuning in to your body to discover how it reacts to exercise to find the adrenal-supporting options that are right for you and ways to slow your breathing to accelerate your healing. I've come to believe that building resilience involves removing inflammatory actions, thoughts, and behaviors, and realizing that our outdated coping mechanisms, resentments, self-limiting beliefs, and trauma may be holding us back from healing and achieving our dreams. You'll find ways to release them, stop tolerating anything that gets your blood boiling or shuts you down, set healthy boundaries, and focus on your goals for living a happy, healthy future. Letting go of what weighs us down makes room for what we do want and creates space for it to manifest.

ATP SUCCESS STORIES

"After taking the ATP, I have less mental fog, less depression, and more compassion for myself. . . . Considering how short [the program] is, I have seen some big improvements in my symptoms. The clarity and focus that [have] come with the program has allowed me to see how my childhood traumas and negative self-talk are causing my immune system to be on high alert. I feel more organized in my life and feel like I have a little more time to work on my self-esteem. Tuning in and using your own abilities to heal yourself is a confidence booster. I feel more love for myself now that I see what I can accomplish."—HOLLY

Review

Tools and quick reference guides, including a schedule for a sample day on the program, distill the key practical takeaways of the protocol so the essentials will always be easy for you to access—and put into action!

Reassess and Move Forward

After completing the fundamental protocols of the ATP, you'll reassess your Adrenal Assessment score from before the start of the program (page 72) to see how it has improved since beginning the interventions and look at potential next steps. For some that may be a maintenance plan, while others may need to dig a little deeper into the root causes of your symptoms to feel 100 percent. I've got you covered! Healing is a journey, not a race, and there are many additional approaches I can share with you to help you on your way.

Chapter 10, "Advanced Stress Symptom Root Causes and Solutions," provides specific interventions to consider to address the top adrenal-related symptoms, such as brain fog and fatigue, insomnia and sleep issues, low libido, mood disturbances (anxiety, depression, overwhelm, irritability, and mood swings), and pain and includes:

- An overview of potential causes and the specific strategies to consider
- Self-directed dietary, supplement, and lifestyle options
- Advanced testing recommendations

After following the ATP, I hope you will be feeling notably better, with higher energy levels and less fatigue, and noticing your symptoms reduce considerably or resolve completely. But if some of your symptoms are lingering, there is still hope and more we can do! Not everyone will need advanced protocols, but if you do, you will find a wealth of ways to keep moving forward on your healing journey.

MY COMMUNITY SPEAKS: THE MOST HELPFUL INTERVENTIONS

According to a recent program survey, the following percentage of participants who filled out the questionnaire found these interventions to be the most helpful:

Intervention	How Many Found It Helpful
Blood Sugar Balance	91%
Hydration	87%
Changing Diet	87%
Simplifying	81%
Self-Compassion	78%
Exercise/Healing Movements	77%
Setting Intentions	74%
Decommitting	74%
Optimizing Sleep	72%
Starting Supplements	72%
Gratitude Journaling	71%
Shifting Thought Patterns and Beliefs	71%
Setting Boundaries	71%

HOW LONG SHOULD THE PROGRAM TAKE?

I've outlined the key elements of the program in the subsequent chapters, and I recommend reading through them, then committing to doing the program for at least four weeks to see the full benefits. Many people may want to continue with the program for more than four weeks, while others will want to add the elements more slowly. Both approaches will work, but please note that all of the interventions work in synergy, so you will see that the benefits of the interventions do build on one another.

If at any point you feel a topic or suggestion is triggering, and you do not have the ability to work through it, please discontinue the activity. If a supplement or way of eating I recommend is not working for you, don't pursue it. A goal of this program is for you and your body to feel safe, and a big part of that is being able to trust your body and your intuition so that you can make the best choices *for you* moving forward.

There's more than one way to peel a potato, as they say, and there's more than one way to heal. As you move through the program, tune in to your body and find the way that works for you. You do not have to follow the program perfectly or do every single strategy to see results, but participants have found that the interventions do work in synergy with one another and doing more of the work usually does translate to more of the results.

Prepare to Take Charge of Your Health

Before you turn to the next chapter and begin the program, I encourage you to take a few steps to prepare yourself for the changes ahead and set the stage for getting better. As you start making significant changes to your lifestyle for healing, it can be very helpful to start a journal dedicated to your healing journey. Use whatever type of journal works best for you. I like a good old-fashioned notebook, but feel free to use your computer, phone, or a journaling app. Your health journal is a place where you can reflect on your goals, set intentions, and create the right mindset.

That's why I created the following exercises and the ones you'll find throughout the program: to help you identify and shift any negative thought patterns you may currently have and reflect on your personal goals. As you take the following steps to take charge of your health, use your journal to reflect on the thoughts and feelings they raise in you as well as record your responses to the "For Reflection" prompts.

You can refer to your responses anytime during the program when you are looking for some motivation, or when you simply need a reminder of why you are committed to your health and to this journey.

Step One: Dream Big (and Write Those Dreams Down!)

Identifying your health goals is the first step in taking charge of your health. If you don't know where you're going, how can you ever get there, right? Setting a goal sets your sights on a desired outcome, concentrates your efforts to achieve it, and gives clear meaning and purpose to the actions you take to make it a reality. It's no surprise then that goal setting is linked to increased self-confidence, motivation, and success. When setting your goals I encourage you to:

Dream Big

Believe in yourself and all that you can accomplish! Whether you want more energy, less pain, refreshing sleep, fewer panic attacks, to be able to keep up with your high-energy toddler (true story), run a 5K, take a spin class, or have a date night, be honest and unafraid to be bold. After all, research suggests that ambitious goals are more motivating than easily achieved ones.

Be Specific

You want to feel better but what exactly does that look like for you? Is there a specific symptom you'd like to eliminate, an activity you'd like to be able to do, or a personal or professional milestone you'd like to achieve? Being as clear and specific as possible makes it easier to track your progress and know if you've succeeded.

Don't edit or judge yourself: No dream is too superficial or silly. If it matters to you, it matters.

Write Them Down

Doing so makes you more likely to achieve your goals. Research by psychologist Gail Matthews showed that people who wrote down their goals were as much as 33 percent more successful in accomplishing them as those who didn't. This may have something to do with how keeping a written record of your goals helps you track your progress and celebrate your successes, increasing the likelihood that you'll attain your goal. And seeing that progress in black and white boosts confidence! Plus, writing down your goals can make you more hopeful and optimistic about the future—and an optimistic outlook contributes to healing.

FOR REFLECTION: DREAM BIG

Start dreaming big by reflecting on the following and writing down your answers. Don't edit or judge your responses. Be honest and as specific as possible. Start creating the future you want for yourself by being crystal clear about what it looks like.

_____

_____

_____

_____

My health goals are:

(Examples: To go to a Pilates class without feeling drained for days. To have enough energy to go out to dinner and a movie with friends. To lose twenty pounds and fit into my favorite jeans. To eliminate my sugar cravings.)

_____

_____

_____

_____

I want to achieve my health goals because:

(Examples: I want to feel beautiful again. I want to be present for my children. I want to shine like I am meant to shine. I want to get a promotion.)

_____

_____

_____

_____

Every time you veer off your path, or feel tempted to, I invite you to come back to these responses, and remind yourself why you are choosing to support your health.

_____

_____

_____

_____

Step Two: Set Your Intentions

As you start making changes to your lifestyle to support your adrenals, another way to foster an optimistic and proactive mindset is to set intentions. Health goals establish where we want to be. Intentions work a little differently. They affirm how we're going to get there. While goals encourage us to look into the future, intentions are rooted in the present moment and how we choose to live or show up in the world right now. They aren't tied to achieving a specific outcome but rather how we act in each moment. Think of an intention as a guiding principle or purpose.

Setting a positive intention at the beginning of your adrenal transformation can help set your thinking and attitude about the changes to come, provide a powerful reminder for how you wish to approach each day, and inspire and motivate you along the way. To create an intention, think about what matters most to you. What would you most like to nurture over the course of the program? How would you most like to experience the next few weeks?

For example:

- I intend to develop a healthier relationship with food.
- I intend to appreciate progress, not perfection.
- I intend to make stress-relieving activities a part of my daily routine.
- I intend to find hope in challenging situations.
- I intend to take advantage of as many of the opportunities for healing in this program as possible.

I truly believe that setting intentions before embarking on a healing journey helps speed up the healing process by putting us in the right mindset. Refer back to them whenever you need a reminder of the commitment you made to yourself at the start of the program. Members who have been stuck on their journey have shared that this practice helps them to feel encouraged and inspired, and that they were finally able to implement the recommendations they knew they needed in order to heal.

FOR REFLECTION: SET YOUR INTENTIONS

How can you show up over the next four weeks to make sure you have the best possible outcome with the program? Consider using this prompt to expand your daily journaling practice and set your intention(s):

I intend to . . .

_____

_____

_____

_____

Step Three: Create Space for Healing

Does it seem like every minute of your day is packed with work, family, and household responsibilities with not a second left over for you? You're not alone. Many of us are more swamped than ever trying to meet the needs of everyone else around us, from kids to significant others, in-laws, and co-workers, leaving us no time for ourselves. Running on empty stresses our adrenals and creates a sense of urgency that prevents resting and healing from happening. And it compromises our ability to care for others. An empty cup cannot fill another. We must fill our own cup first.

Getting the most from the program means investing in yourself and finding more time for self-care. The people who have the best results set aside some time every day to prepare for the week ahead, write in their health journal, de-stress, and rest. This is a special time to give your health your full attention.

You're probably wondering, *How can I do all of this when time is already so tight?* You can find a lot more space in each day by making time- and energy-sucking tasks more efficient—or eliminating them completely! Remember the last time you ran out of toilet paper and had to go racing to the store at rush hour for a roll? Or had to dash out to the post office for stamps to pay your bills? You may not think these errands take up a lot of time, but they really do, and it adds up quickly.

Take a closer look at the tasks that keep you busy throughout the day. What can you:

- **Eliminate:** Is this a task you could get out of your way by deciding it's time to just say no?
- **Simplify:** Could the process be streamlined?
- **Automate:** Could you use a service, app, or other technology to execute recurring tasks?
- **Delegate:** Could you assign responsibility or partial responsibility to someone else and take on a more supervisory role?

Once you start looking for redundancies and inefficiencies in your routines, you'll discover how much low-hanging fruit there is to pick! As an entrepreneur, mom, and somebody trying to make space in my life for healing, I'm always looking for potential opportunities to save some time. These are my top ten suggestions for freeing up precious time and energy for self-care:

1. Keep a reserve of nonperishable items like toilet paper and paper towels or order them through a recurring subscription.

2. Have medications on automatic refill or delivered to your house, to save yourself a trip to the pharmacy.

3. Just the same, some companies offer for your supplements to be renewed automatically, and mailed to you each month, so you don't have to spend time reordering them.

4. Set your bills to "automatic payment."

5. Use on-demand and subscription grocery, grass-fed, pasture-raised animal protein, and wild-caught/organic seafood delivery services to avoid multiple visits to the store.

6. Assign household chores to family members or hire someone to clean your home or parts of your home, such as the floors and bathrooms.

7. Identify at least one backup caregiver for your children or pets to avoid scrambling for care at the last minute if your primary caregiver is unavailable.

8. Limit your availability by phone, text, email, and social media. Use your phone's "do not disturb" function or silence individual app notifications. To get your social media apps "out of sight, out of mind," place all of them in their own folder, away from your main screen. Try it out. You will be surprised by how many times you may reach for your phone for the first few days!

9. Check emails at designated times each day instead of checking them all day long.

10. Consider meal plan services to make eating a healthy diet less time consuming. Alternately, instead of cooking each day, you can batch cook and meal prep multiple portions of food for a few hours each week—less cleanup and more food, and thus a huge timesaver!

There are always tasks that can be eliminated, simplified, automated, or delegated. Having fewer commitments on your plate, especially in the evenings, can allow you to go to bed at a reasonably early time . . . and not feel guilty about it. If you are feeling overwhelmed, reflect on areas in your life that you can work on. For example, are you being bombarded by extra job responsibilities? If so, speak up and see if you can delegate some of your tasks to others! Do you have too many social obligations, is your schedule jam-packed with volunteer work, or have you offered one too many favors lately? Don't be afraid to say no and turn down a few, or reschedule some commitments for another time. Remember, self-care is just as important as caring for others and essential for taking back your health.

Step Four: Practice Gratitude

My mentor, JJ Virgin, taught me that one of the fastest ways to overcome overwhelm is through practicing gratitude. I invite you to acknowledge the goodness in your life. There is always something to be grateful for: waking up in the morning, your nice smile, the laughter of your children, a thoughtful email from a friend, the flowers in your garden, the refreshing sweetness of a fresh berry, the feel of soft, clean sheets against your skin, the playful antics of your dog. Practicing gratitude by regularly noticing and being thankful for the special people, moments, and experiences that surround us is one of the quickest ways to make ourselves feel better and keep us motivated. A 2020 study review found that gratitude practices led to individuals experiencing improved sleep quality, as well as improved physical health markers such as blood pressure, blood sugar regulation, and asthma. Another study found that those who practice gratitude feel less stressed.

Each day of the program, I encourage you to take a few minutes and cultivate a positive outlook by writing down three things you are grateful for.

Today I am grateful for:
1.
2.
3.

I love this practice and try to do it on a regular basis. Some days, I practice gratitude by sending emails, messages, or thank-you notes to people for whom I am grateful. Try this, too. You can also send yourself gratitude notes or buy yourself gratitude gifts.

However you choose to express your gratitude for others and yourself, make being thankful a part of your routine. Giving thanks in the coming weeks will help you appreciate all of the efforts you are making to restore your health and work through any challenges when they arise.

With an attitude of gratitude, cravings were no match for Laura P., who shared: "*Wow*, I am feeling really good on this diet. Loving myself through the sugar cravings . . . keeping in mind to easy does it and just enjoy each moment with gratitude!" Gratitude can be your superpower, too.

Step Five: Validate Your Situation—and Get Ready for Action

No matter what you're feeling about your situation right now—sadness, anger, fear, confusion, frustration—I want you to know it's okay and perfectly normal. Be kind and gentle with yourself, showing the same amount of compassion you would have for a loved one. Allow yourself to feel and express these emotions rather than suppress them. Repressed emotions have been linked to lower immune system function, stress, and anxiety, none of which I've found to be helpful for healing.

Give yourself the time and space to work through these emotions but be careful not to drift into indefinite wallowing. Spending too much time feeling sorry for yourself will prevent you from taking the actions necessary to help you get better. A 2012 study from Case Western Reserve University found that empathy and logical thinking turn off each other. This means that if you're feeling sorry for yourself, you may not make the best logical decisions for your health—or any decisions at all.

I know it can be difficult to approach your condition objectively, but once you've taken the time to grieve, I encourage you to start thinking like an objective scientist or care manager, implementing strategies, monitoring results, and adjusting as needed along the way. Direct your energy and efforts toward getting better, and it will happen.

How Are You Doing? No Really, How Are You?

I grew up in Poland and moved to the United States when I was nine years old. It wasn't until I was almost twenty-five years old that I learned that when English speakers ask the question "How are you?" they don't actually want to know! I remember this coming as a big shock. When I was working as a consulting pharmacist for a case management agency, a social worker (we'll call him Bob) came into my office to ask for guidance regarding medications one of his clients was taking. Bob knocked on my office door and said, "Dr. Wentz, how are you?" I proceeded to tell him that I was a little bit tired because my dog had kept me awake the previous night, and let's just say this gentleman did not have much of a poker face. Bob looked at me with a very confused grin and said, "Okay, well anyway . . ." In Western societies, "How are you?" is often used as a greeting, and the expected answer is always "Okay," "Great," or "Good," followed by a polite "And how are you?"

In a similar fashion, many of us are taught to suppress our feelings (often from an early age, as children who are told that they are "okay" after a painful fall by parents who are uncomfortable with sad feelings), and we often miss the early signs that we may not be okay, great, or good. We tend to minimize our symptoms for fear of being labeled crybabies, hypochondriacs,

---

TRY JOURNALING EACH DAY

In addition to using your health journal to reflect on the exercises provided throughout the *Adrenal Transformation Protocol*, I encourage you to develop your own daily journaling practice to help you process your journey and find inspiration along the way.

Here is a list of journal prompts I encourage you to work with:

- How I feel today
- Today's healing affirmation (I love myself; I am healing)
- Three things I am grateful for
- What time I went to bed, what time I woke up this morning, how my quality of sleep was
- Self-care notes
- What I learned today/reflection

I developed a special journal to support you on your healing journey and inspire you to write in it regularly. You can see it on page 68. Feel free to model or modify your own journaling based on these prompts. If you would like to download a printable version of this journal, go to thyroidpharmacist.com/atpbookbonus.

Date:_____

Today I am grateful for:

How I feel today:

Today's healing affirmation:

Time to bed:

Time awake:

Quality of sleep:

Self-care notes:

What I learned today/reflection:

and worse. Adding to the insult, many people with chronic illness spend years being gaslighted by their doctors who deny their symptoms. For these reasons, many of us suffer alone.

At this time, I give you permission to take an honest inventory of your symptoms. In order to heal, and to determine if the interventions you are making are helping you, let's figure out where you are right now.

I've included the questionnaire below so that you can determine your current adrenal stress score and keep track of your progress as you follow the guidance in the four-week program. I recommend bookmarking this page and checking in with your body after each week of doing the program.

The Adrenal Assessment

I encourage you to take an honest inventory of how you feel before you start any health improvement program. This will let you see if the program is helping. In the chart below, please rate the symptoms that apply to you with a score of 0–10, 0 meaning the symptom is not present and 10 meaning the symptom is severe.

Mark the score for each symptom that applies to you currently in the section called "baseline." You will come back to this assessment at the end of each week of the four-week program to mark your progress.

You will notice that your symptom scores will reduce each week and then altogether disappear after you complete the entire four-week program detailed in Part II of the book.

We will address any remaining symptoms in Part III with the Advanced Protocols.

THYROID TIP

If you have a thyroid condition, I recommend working with your physician to monitor your thyroid function every six to twelve weeks while making lifestyle changes. As you heal your adrenals, you may find that you utilize your thyroid medications better, so we want to watch your levels to make sure you don't become overmedicated.

Symptom	Baseline	After Week 1	After Week 2	After Week 3	After Week 4
I feel fatigued.					
I have brain fog or trouble remembering things.					
I feel emotional and have trouble managing my emotions.					
I feel anxious, worried, or nervous.					
I have panic attacks.					
I feel depressed, moody, or sad.					
I have pain, such as cramps, joint pain, or muscle pain.					
My muscles feel weak.					
I have sleep problems (either falling asleep or staying asleep).					
I have nonrestorative sleep (I don't feel reenergized).					
I feel stressed most of the time.					
I feel tired but wired.					
I have low blood pressure (less than 120/80 mmHg).					
I feel dizzy when I stand up.					
I have hypoglycemia (low blood sugar).					
I get irritable when I skip meals or go too long without eating.					

Symptom	Baseline	After Week 1	After Week 2	After Week 3	After Week 4
I crave salt.					
I startle easily.					
I have morning fatigue.					
I often feel overwhelmed.					
I have low libido.					
I often feel irritable.					
I crave sweets.					
I have dark circles under my eyes.					
I have mental fogginess or trouble concentrating.					
I have headaches or migraines.					
I have frequent infections (I catch cold easily).					
I don't tolerate exercise well and feel completely exhausted afterward.					
I retain water.					
I have heart palpitations.					
I need to start the day with caffeine.					
I have poor tolerance to alcohol, caffeine, and other drugs.					
I feel weak and shaky.					
I have sweaty palms and feet when nervous.					

Symptom	Baseline	After Week 1	After Week 2	After Week 3	After Week 4
I feel too hot and struggle with heat intolerance.					
I have night sweats.					
I have hair loss.					
I feel too cold or have cold intolerance.					
I can't lose weight despite efforts.					
I can't gain weight despite efforts.					
I have acne.					
I have acid reflux.					
I have diarrhea or constipation.					
It takes me longer to heal.					
I am indecisive.					
Total Number of Symptoms Present					
Total Score					

No matter where you fall on this assessment right now, please know that completing this program can make you feel beautiful, fit, calm, and healthy, and you are the one who will make it happen!

You'll retake the assessment at the end of each week you are on the program to see how many of your symptoms have gone away or improved.

We might start off with twenty symptoms and nineteen of them go away, but being human, we might focus on that one symptom that's left and forget to celebrate all of our successes. I really want to make sure that throughout this program you celebrate yourself and your progress, because every change is a step toward healing!

SIGNS OF ACUTE ADRENAL FAILURE OR ADDISONIAN CRISIS

While most people with adrenal dysfunction do not have Addison's disease, I do want to caution you about the signs and symptoms indicating Addison's disease or damaged adrenals that are unable to produce enough cortisol, just in case they align with your current condition. If so, it's important to seek emergency medical treatment. Dangerously low levels of cortisol can be life-threatening.

- Extreme weakness
- Mental confusion
- Dizziness
- Vomiting
- Fever
- Sudden pain in your lower back or legs
- Nausea or severe abdominal pain
- Extremely low blood pressure
- Reduced consciousness or delirium

Strange but True Physical Signs of Adrenal Dysfunction

In addition to looking at your symptoms, you can determine if you have adrenal dysfunction by utilizing the following self-assessments.

- **Are you irritable?** Irritability and overwhelm are two cardinal signs of adrenal dysfunction. My best test for determining adrenal issues is being snappy or short-tempered, feeling overwhelmed, or finding other people annoying. For example, I can always tell that my adrenals are overwhelmed when my mom calls to say hello, and I feel like it is too much of a demand to talk to her!
- **Do you have low blood pressure?** People with adrenal dysfunction often have low blood pressure and/or a drop in blood pressure after

standing up from a lying-down or sitting position (orthostatic hypotension). They may also experience dizziness or light-headedness when changing positions. A great way to test for this is by measuring your blood pressure while lying down, then standing up and measuring your blood pressure again. This is a common test functional doctors perform to determine the adrenal function of a patient. An individual is classified as having orthostatic hypotension if there is a significant decrease in blood pressure within three minutes of standing up. For example, a decrease of blood pressure from 120/80 to 90/60 is a significant one that may mean that your adrenals are underactive or that you are dehydrated.

- **Do you have light sensitivity?** People with low adrenal function may often have difficulty contracting their pupils. Usually our pupils dilate (enlarge) in the dark and contract (get smaller) in the light. Symptoms of adrenal dysfunction may include light sensitivity, difficulty seeing in bright lights, having to wear sunglasses on most days, or, as I like to call it, feeling like a vampire in daylight!

- **Is your body temperature unstable?** If you are keeping track of your first morning temperatures for fertility tracking, morning temperatures that are fluctuating and on the low side may be suggestive of adrenal insufficiency. You may have heard that low temperatures are a sign of an underactive thyroid, and this is correct as well. Hypothyroidism or an underactive thyroid will also present as low temperatures, but the low temperatures will be daily and stable.

- **Do you crave the whole bag of chips?** Have you ever eaten (or wanted to eat) an entire bag of chips in one sitting? You're not alone! Salt cravings are a cardinal sign of adrenal issues (along with feeling "salty," of course!). With adrenal issues, we may find ourselves with intense cravings for salty foods like crackers, chips, pretzels, and olives.

- **Do you sometimes feel "hangry"?** If you skip a meal, or go too long without eating, do you become angry or irritable? That irritable, tantrum-throwing child of hunger and anger is named "Hangry," and I would not recommend having her over for a playdate.

WHAT IT FEELS LIKE TO HAVE ADRENAL DYSFUNCTION

A list of clinical symptoms can never really quite capture what it feels like to live with adrenal dysfunction. I asked my Facebook community to share their experiences in their own words in the hope of helping you feel more understood and less alone—and assure you that no matter the darkness you feel right now, you can get better and get your life back. I've done it, and thousands of my clients and readers have, too. Here are some of their comments:

"I have absolutely no energy upon waking, sleep 8+ hours and still feel as if I need 8+ more hours of sleep, and feel as if there are cement blocks strapped to my feet. I have irrational feelings of sadness, jealousy, and anger, oftentimes unprovoked and unreasonable. I forget dates, thoughts mid-sentence, and why I walked into a room."

"One day I have lots of energy and feel like doing but the next day I am down and out with no energy at all. The hardest part is having the to-do list in my brain and wanting to get it all done but my body says otherwise."

"I'll wake up in the middle of the night with the physiological presentation of anxiety but not the mental preoccupation. It feels like a massive sugar rush at 3 a.m. when I've not eaten anything or had any caffeine."

"I'm 56 and sometimes feel like my 85-year-old mother can outdo me in just about everything in everyday life."

"Felt like falling apart; was uncomfortable to leave the house. . . . Am I safe? Am I gonna die?"

"As if all of the energy is being sucked from my body, a physical and mental crash, directly following any small stressful event (even an argument with my teen to clean her room). Constant brain fog plagues me daily as well. I toss and turn all night. Forget about exercise . . . I lose all physical strength almost instantly."

"You are wired but tired. Exercise that is supposed to give you more energy takes it all away. . . . A little stress will take all your energy away. . . . You are completely drained to the point where you can't talk or socialize with anyone for days. It's isolating, people don't understand you."

"I frequently felt this panicky feeling like I needed to bolt and run as fast as I can, away from the stress (flight response)."

"I felt 'pregnant tired' but I wasn't pregnant. And had to drink so much caffeine to barely make it through the day and even then I sometimes couldn't keep myself awake all day. . . . Trying to think felt like trying to wade through mud."

"Feeling overwhelmed at the simplest of things. Minor decisions seem epic and I tend to panic some days just trying to decide what pair of shoes to wear! I used to manage extreme amounts of stress like a champ but my body has shut that down. Then lack of sleep just exacerbates it. But there are good days too. My adrenal issues have taught me how to listen more intuitively to my body and to prioritize myself finally. I am gentler and kinder to my body now. I have to be."

"I can't handle the tiniest of stress anymore. Everyone thinks I'm being a drama queen."

I've found that symptom self-assessments like these and the Adrenal Assessment questionnaire are excellent indicators of an impaired stress response and provide the information we need to start providing the body with the right kind of support. That's why, as I mentioned earlier, the ATP is designed to work without medical testing. I want to empower you to understand your own body and what it needs, without the reliance on tests. If I can teach you just one thing with this book, it is to remember to listen to your body, as your body is wise and powerful. By tuning in to your symptoms, you can determine where your body is and what it needs.

So let's listen even more closely! By paying a little more attention to your body and the timing of the symptoms you are experiencing, you can pretty accurately figure out which stage of adrenal dysfunction you are in and tailor certain nutrition and supplement protocols to your unique situation. Let's take a closer look at the optimal release pattern of cortisol throughout the day and what your symptoms are telling us about your current pattern.

Assessing Your Adrenal Health: From Optimal to Advanced Dysfunction

Optimally functioning adrenals are supposed to put out the most cortisol in the morning, and the levels of cortisol should decline gradually and smoothly during the day, until very little cortisol is secreted at bedtime. A cortisol kick in the morning helps us to get out of bed bright-eyed and bushy-tailed, ready to face the day. Low cortisol secretion at bedtime helps us unwind, relax, and sleep.

Please see the image below. Do you notice how the black line follows the gray, optimal range curve? This is what I would consider to be a beautiful, optimal cortisol curve of a person who wakes up with great energy in the morning; feels calm, happy, and productive during the day; and has an easy time winding down at bedtime, falling asleep, and staying asleep. This person is thriving, and you can get there too after completing this program. ☺

NORMAL ADRENAL FUNCTION

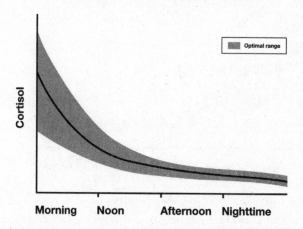

When cortisol levels are not aligned with this pattern, we have very predictable symptoms. People with adrenal dysfunction can have three different patterns, and the patterns are progressive, starting with a high-cortisol stage, followed by a cortisol roller-coaster stage, and ending at cortisol deficiency.

Stage I: High-Cortisol Stage

In this initial stage, the HPA axis is over-responsive, with high total cortisol. Excess cortisol all day long, including in the evening when levels should be low to allow us to fall asleep, causes many people to feel anxious, irritable, restless, and wired (but tired) during the day.

Additionally, while it may not be felt, this high level of cortisol breaks down the body, leading to joint and muscle pain, sleeplessness, sugar cravings, low sex drive, and digestive distress. (Think of a bunch of rock stars on uppers in a shabby little hotel room, partying on all cylinders, not realizing that they are destroying everything in sight—including their own bodies.)

Unless an intervention is made to address this, the body will progress to Stage II, to protect itself from the damaging effects of excess cortisol. In my experience, people are often too busy to seek help in this stage, or mostly look to conventional medicine for help, and receive "Band-Aids" such as pain medications, sedatives for sleep, Viagra-like pills, and acid-suppressing medications.

STAGE 1 OF ADRENAL DYSFUNCTION

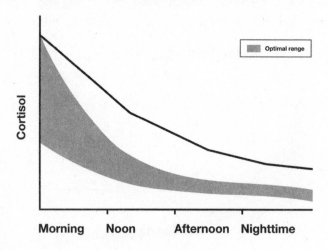

Stage II: Cortisol Roller-Coaster Stage

The body gets into a protective mode, and the communication breakdown between the brain and adrenals starts to develop. The body is still under stress, but as in "The Boy Who Cried Wolf," the same emergency response is not launched each time stress is perceived.

Overall cortisol levels are normal, but there are fluctuations in the cortisol rhythm, such as excessively low cortisol in the morning and too much later in the day. With this flipped pattern, people may have a hard time getting up in the morning and drag their feet until the early afternoon.

They will feel more energetic in the afternoon but will grow a bit anxious as the day progresses and will feel slightly human until about 8 p.m. Just before they're ready to go to sleep, they will hit a second wind. They are alert and sleepy at the wrong times, leading to poor energy levels, anxiety, and trouble sleeping.

This curve looks a bit like a roller coaster, and the people riding this curve often report that they are on an emotional roller coaster and may be prescribed medications for mood disorders, anxiety, or depression. More people are likely to seek help from integrative medicine at this point, but unfortunately, as the total cortisol is "normal" on testing, this dysfunctional pattern is often misunderstood and considered normal by practitioners new to integrative medicine and by patients who run and interpret their own cortisol saliva labs.

STAGE 2 OF ADRENAL DYSFUNCTION

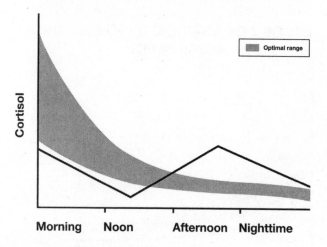

Stage III: Cortisol Deficiency Stage

The final and most advanced stage of adrenal dysfunction is the low-cortisol stage, known as hypercortisolism. Total cortisol is low, all day, every day. At this stage, there is a complete breakdown of the communication pathways.

Naturopathic doctors used to say that the adrenals were fatigued and couldn't make more cortisol. But that's not necessarily the case. Can the adrenals make more cortisol? Sure. But are they going to? No. They don't feel like it. This is because they are no longer responding to the signals from the pituitary.

People in this advanced stage of adrenal dysfunction are often tired all day long. They wake up tired, they sludge through most of the day, and they go to sleep tired.

At this point, many people's bodies have not had enough time to repair, have run out of nutrients that are required for repair, and they are often diagnosed with chronic fatigue or some sort of autoimmune, inflammatory condition that ends in "itis" (arthritis, thyroiditis).

This is the dysfunction pattern of most people I have worked with. In my experience, people at this stage have often been to numerous doctors and received little help. This is where I was when I first discovered I had adrenal dysfunction, and I can tell you that it's not fun. Luckily, regardless of where you may fall on this curve, I can help.

In the early stages, the cortisol starts to drop beneath the gray, optimal range.

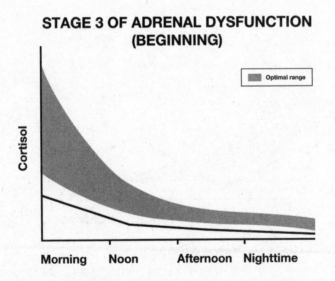

STAGE 3 OF ADRENAL DYSFUNCTION (BEGINNING)

As time goes on, the cortisol drops lower and lower (unless an intervention is made), and people end up becoming exhausted and often caffeine dependent. They may be diagnosed with chronic fatigue syndrome, fibromyalgia, Hashimoto's, or another autoimmune inflammatory condition, as cortisol is too low to balance the unchecked inflammation. As you can tell, the curve has mostly lost its shape at this point and looks more like a line. I refer to this advanced stage of adrenal dysfunction as "flatlined" adrenals.

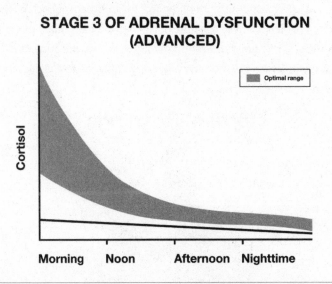

STAGE 3 OF ADRENAL DYSFUNCTION (ADVANCED)

Cortisol

Optimal range

Morning   Noon   Afternoon   Nighttime

LOW CORTISOL BY THE STATS

While much of what you may hear on the news regarding cortisol focuses on excess cortisol being "bad," low cortisol can be even worse, and cortisol that is produced at the wrong times can be really ugly, in terms of causing a lot of irritability and anxiety (the "I just yelled at everyone" kind).

In my client work, I have primarily worked with people with Hashimoto's or some sort of autoimmune condition. When people's health has declined to the point when they have an autoimmune condition, they have progressed from a cortisol excess, the beginning stage of adrenal dysfunction, into an advanced stage of adrenal dysfunction where their daily cortisol output is too low.

In analyzing 148 adrenal saliva tests of symptomatic people with Hashimoto's from 2015 to 2019, I have noticed that all of the individuals tested had some degree of adrenal dysfunction.

While 7 out of 148 tested individuals showed an excess of cortisol, 91 individuals had low levels of cortisol. Furthermore, of the 50 people whose cortisol was in the "normal range," their cortisol curve was off: they were producing either too little cortisol in the morning; they had fluctuations at their noon/afternoon readings; or they produced too much at night, leading to morning fatigue, midday mood swings, and/ or trouble sleeping at night.

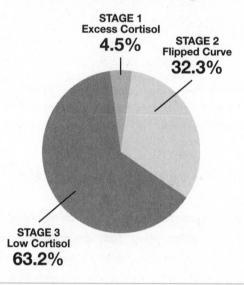

Cortisol Readings

STAGE 1
Excess Cortisol
4.5%

STAGE 2
Flipped Curve
32.3%

STAGE 3
Low Cortisol
63.2%

Do You Need an Adrenal Test?

I have analyzed hundreds of these adrenal cortisol curves, and when the test is done by a reputable lab that utilizes the correct reference ranges, I was able to accurately predict the clients' exact symptoms throughout the day, simply by looking at their cortisol curves. As time went on, the adrenal lab testing company I was using, BioHealth, redefined their reference ranges, and the test results no longer matched the clients' experience.

I decided to try interpreting the tests using the lab's old reference ranges, and lo and behold, this allowed for precise interpretation of symptoms once more. However, the company went out of business in 2019.

I used to teach my clients and the participants of my Hashimoto's Self-Management Program about how to order and interpret their own adrenal tests, but not all lab tests are created equally, and things can change. And as I've mentioned, I want to empower you to understand your own body and what it needs, without the reliance on tests.

Through reviewing hundreds of adrenal saliva labs, I've isolated very specific symptoms that can predict your cortisol levels.

So while adrenal saliva and urine tests can be super helpful to determine the precise stage of adrenal dysfunction, you do not need one to begin the ATP. Rather, I will share how to tune in to your symptoms in order to determine whether you are experiencing high cortisol, low cortisol, or the cortisol roller coaster.

Circle your symptoms on the chart below to determine whether you have more symptoms of cortisol deficiency or excess cortisol.

WHAT ARE YOUR SYMPTOMS OF CORTISOL DYSREGULATION?

Having too little or too much cortisol can cause a range of symptoms. Tuning in to your symptoms can guide you as to whether you have low cortisol and need to emphasize cortisol-boosting activities (like bright lights* and certain foods and supplements) and avoid cortisol-lowering activities (like aerobic exercise and certain supplements), or have high cortisol and need to prioritize cortisol-lowering activities and skip cortisol boosters.

	Cortisol Deficiency All Day	Excess Cortisol All Day
I feel	Wiped out, tired all day	Anxious, racing thoughts, edgy, high-strung, and unable to relax
Blood sugar is	Low, may have hypoglycemia	High

	Cortisol Deficiency All Day	Excess Cortisol All Day
Blood pressure is	Low or borderline low, or drops when I get up (you feel faint when standing too quickly) (less than 120/80 mmHg)	High or borderline high (above 120/80 mmHg)
Muscles are	Weak, tired, achy	Tense and tight, achy
Hydration	Dehydration, due to increased thirst and frequency of urination	More likely to have water retention, due to cortisol's increase of antidiuretic hormone
Aerobic exercise makes me feel	More tired	More relaxed and balanced
Sleep	Even if I fall asleep easily, my sleep is unrefreshing	Difficulty with falling asleep
Count How Many Symptoms You Have in Each Column	Cortisol Deficiency _____5_____	Cortisol Excess _____

*bright lights should follow a circadian pattern, lots of light in the morning, darkness at night

How to Tell If Your Symptoms Are Due to Low or High Cortisol

- Count up the symptoms you have in each column.
- If all or most of your symptoms fall on the left column of the chart, there's a good chance that you have low cortisol.
- If all or most of your symptoms fall on the right column of the chart, there's a good chance that you have high cortisol.
- Individuals who find themselves with some symptoms of high cortisol and some symptoms of low cortisol and/or report feeling a sense of overwhelm, difficulty staying asleep, erratic mental function, and feeling like they are on an emotional roller coaster are likely to be in Stage II of adrenal dysfunction.

- If you still don't have a full resolution of your symptoms by the end of the program, I'll share some additional strategies to help you reach your goals, which may include lab tests.

  Most of the strategies that are covered in the program will help you no matter which stage you are in by addressing the underlying reasons for cortisol dysregulation and supporting the consequences of those cortisol alterations so you can feel balanced once more. For those individuals who identify with having high or low cortisol, I have included a few specific strategies for your unique situation, which you will find within the relevant chapters.

Kick Off Your Healing

It's okay if you feel overwhelmed after taking these assessments and realizing just how many symptoms you're dealing with. I want to remind you that you are already taking steps to turn these symptoms around. Thousands of others have healed their adrenals with my protocols, which has allowed them to regain their health. You can, too. In the next chapters, I'm going to guide you on the steps you need to take to help eliminate your stress symptoms and to create a sense of safety in your body so that you can feel strong, calm, powerful, and full of energy.

In my online group program, we go on this journey together, and the participants receive daily reminders of action steps to take. We see a lot of symptoms reported at baseline, and during week 1, but right around week 2, we start seeing a big shift, followed by further improvements by weeks 3 and 4. So please know that you can get better, but it will take some work, and perhaps some planning on your end. I hope this book will give you the knowledge and power to take back your health.

If We Fail to Plan, We Plan to Fail

If we fail to plan, we plan to fail. As you read the subsequent chapters, I encourage you to pick a start date for when you will implement the diet, supplements, and lifestyle changes, and give the diet and supplements at least three weeks to work.

I know lifestyle changes can be tough, and sometimes it helps to break them down into small goals. In some cases, you may be able to achieve numerous goals in one day; in other cases, one goal may take a few days to complete.

You may wish to read all of Part II and the recipes before diving in, and give yourself a week or two to prepare yourself for doing the program.

I do recommend starting with the diet, supplements, and oxytocin-boosting healing modalities in Chapters 4, 5, and 6 before jumping into building resilience with the strength-training exercises and personal transformational work in Chapter 7. Here's a sample schedule I share with my group coaching clients that you can follow. Feel free to write in a target date for yourself in the "Date Completed" column. Remember to refer back to this schedule to help keep you on track during the four weeks.

Sample Schedule for the Four-Week Program

Date Completed	Focus	Page Number
	Review Part II of *Adrenal Transformation Protocol*	91
	Start Health/Gratitude Journal	66–68
	Set Intentions	61
	Review Supplement Summary and Order Supplements	247
	Review Recipes and Shop for Ingredients	295
	Create Space for Healing	62
	Baseline Symptom Check-In	70

Week 1 Plan

Date Completed	Focus	Page Number
	Start Your Healing Diet	91
	Better/Worse Inventory	185
	Mindset	59

Date Completed	Focus	Page Number
	Add Strategies That Create Safety and Boost Oxytocin	185
	Circadian Balance: Get More Sleep	168
	Week 1 Symptom Check-In	70

Week 2 Plan

Date Completed	Focus	Page Number
	Set Up Supplements	247
	Start Your Supplements!	247
	Hydration and Electrolytes	151
	Circadian Balance: Bright Daytime Lights	169
	Meditation	211
	Balancing Teas	159
	Caffeine Wean (optional)	158
	Week 2 Symptom Check-In	70

Week 3 Plan

Date Completed	Focus	Page Number
	Affirmations	180
	Get Creative	199
	Self-Compassion	179
	Create Your Trigger Toolkit	214
	Forgiveness	226
	Week 3 Symptom Check-In	70

Week 4 Plan

Date Completed	Focus	Page Number
	Self-Limiting Beliefs	231
	Traumas	234

leted	Focus	Page Number
	Boundaries	236
	Stop Tolerating	230
	Feel-Good Movement	206
	Week 4 Symptom Check-In	70

After Completing the Four-Week Program

Date Completed	Focus	Page Number
	Read Part III of *Adrenal Transformation Protocol*	255–292
	Plan Next Healing Steps	255
	Troubleshoot Remaining Symptoms: Look into Specific Symptom Solutions	267

Chapter 3 Essentials for Your Journey

- Follow the ATP to send your body safety signals, address the top chronic stressors sabotaging your adrenals, and build resilience throughout your body.
- If you're still experiencing anxiety, irritability, brain fog, fatigue, pain, libido issues, and other top adrenal-related symptoms after completing the program for at least four weeks, turn to Chapter 10, "Advanced Stress Symptom Root Causes and Solutions," for additional root cause interventions aimed at healing the symptoms still troubling you and helping you get to 100 percent.
- Kick off your healing by taking the Adrenal Assessment, listening to your body to determine which cortisol pattern aligns with your symptoms, reviewing the sample schedule, and setting a start date to begin the program—making sure to allow enough time to adequately prepare!
- Turn the page to begin your transformation!

To view the scientific references cited in this chapter, please visit us online at https://thyroidpharmacist.com/atpbooknotes.

PART II

The Adrenal Transformation Protocol

CHAPTER 4

Replenish

Goals

- Learn why eating nutritious food sends safety signals to our bodies.
- Use food and targeted supplementation to rebalance the stress response and accelerate your healing.
- Eat the right things at the right times to eliminate blood sugar swings.
- Start building healthier habits that your body will thank you for for years to come!

Welcome to the ATP! You are going to experience so many wonderful changes and you will start to release those heavy symptoms you've been carrying with you. You will discover ways to send safety signals to your body to promote healing and build resilience. As your symptoms start to vanish, you'll feel lighter, brighter, and less stressed. Each day over the course of this four-week program, you'll take one step closer to the person you are meant to be.

I've said it once, and I'll say it time and time again: Nutrition is one of the most powerful ways to send the body safety signals. In this chapter, I'm going to share three key ways to send safety signals and rebalance your adrenal stress response using nutrition.

1. **Nutrient density:** When we are depleted of nutrients, whether micronutrients (like vitamins and minerals) or macronutrients (like fats and proteins), or simply have a caloric deficit or don't eat at regular intervals, the body receives the message that food is scarce and that we are in a famine. We will send the message of nutrient density by eating

more nutrient-rich and nourishing foods, forgoing processed foods, eating at frequent intervals, eating until full, and supplementing with nutrients that are commonly depleted by the stress response as well as nourishing and balancing adaptogenic herbs.

2. **Lowered inflammation:** Inflammation can contribute to the body's perception of danger. We will address dietary sources of inflammation by eliminating inflammatory foods, including food sensitivities, and addressing a major internal source of inflammation, an unbalanced microbiome in the gut, with probiotic foods and the probiotic supplement *Saccharomyces boulardii.*

3. **Balanced blood sugar:** Blood sugar swings lead to a release of our stress hormones, while blood sugar balance provides hormonal stability that translates to mood stability and a sense of calmness. We will help the body to feel safe by eating for blood sugar balance and utilizing two important blood sugar–balancing supplements: myo-inositol and carnitine.

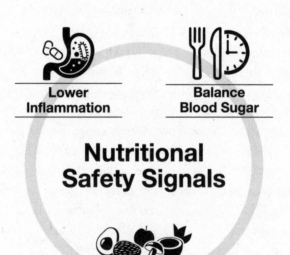

Nutritional Safety Signals

Lower Inflammation

Balance Blood Sugar

Nutrient Density

Replenishing with Food

The world of nutrition is full of competing messages: Some experts recommend calorie-restricted diets, fasting, juicing, and vegan/vegetarian diets as the key to health; other food plans, like the Paleo, carnivore, and ketogenic diets, are centered around meat, high-fat dairy, and/or lower carbohydrates. Then there is the camp that says "diets" are completely worthless and that cutting out any food is a sign of an eating disorder! The extensive marketing of weight-loss diets, grocery stores packed with cheap processed foods, and our reliance on the Standard American Diet (SAD)—an appropriate acronym—cause stress and disease. Flavor enhancers and additives actually trick our brains and palates into thinking we want or need that food!

Marketing messages and mass-produced food are not only confusing and unhealthy; they steer us away from the kind of eating that we should be doing: eating plenty of nourishing, whole foods and stepping away from foods that our bodies know they don't want. When we filter out all of those marketing messages and learn to just listen to our bodies, everything is simpler. We reduce physiological stress and send safety signals to our bodies.

When I think of eating for adrenal balance, I like to think of a cavewoman (or cave person!) who has only her own intuition (and non-processed food) to work with. She eats food that really makes her feel good, instead of food that would cause stomachaches, bloating, or lethargy. She eats until she is full and drinks to satisfy her thirst with adequate water and electrolytes. Without artificial lights and online streaming services, she eats during daylight hours and enjoys deep rest at night, instead of binging on movies and pizza after dark and lying awake for hours (let me tell you, I've been there, done that, and would not recommend it).

Eating foods that make you feel good and limiting foods that make you feel bad will help you heal. Now if you are anything like I was at the beginning of my healing journey, you're probably thinking, *I already eat foods that make me feel good, and don't eat anything that makes me feel bad.* For some, potato chips, cookies, and ice cream are "feel-good foods," and I've also worked with many people who have identified as "the healthiest sick person they knew," because they really try to eat plenty of foods that are conventionally considered to be healthy, such as grains and low-fat dairy. But here's the thing: When we have chronic symptoms, the connection to foods may be difficult to pinpoint. This is because when we react to foods we are constantly eating, the body may not readily let us know that we are reacting to something right away. Rather, inflammatory foods most often cause a delayed reaction that can take hours to days to manifest. Thus the feedback loop, and our body's wisdom, is disconnected from the foods we eat. We will need to reestablish this feedback mechanism by taking at least three weeks to eat an unprocessed diet, free of the most common reactive foods. People who have tried the ATP diet will report that they usually see improvements within three to five days (although symptoms may take longer to vanish fully), and that reintroducing a food after at least twenty-one days of abstaining will result in a much easier way to identify inflammatory reaction.

So . . . what does our cavewoman subsist on? Whole, unprocessed foods that can be eaten raw or cooked without fancy processing, including fruits, vegetables, proteins, eggs, nuts, and seeds—the foods that are hunted and gathered, not the foods that are processed or milled, like baguettes or grains, and no, cavewomen did not have access to frozen yogurt, or even cows for that matter. Sound familiar? Yes, the foods she would have eaten are similar to today's Paleo diet. I recommend this diet because it minimizes inflammatory foods, emphasizes nutrient-rich foods, supports stable blood sugar, and is easy to follow.

I had been recommending the Paleo diet for people with Hashimoto's and other health challenges for close to a decade when I released the ATP. When surveying ATP members before and after the program, 93 percent of those who implemented all of the dietary changes reported that the changes were helpful, and 100 percent of people who specifically tried the blood sugar–balancing recommendations said that they were helpful! As one participant, Tabitha K., shared: "I think the diet changes gave me the most noticeable improvement. . . . After the first week with the diet changes I could tell a difference. I feel like the version of me from over 20 years ago. . . . I have lost weight and inflammation in my joints."

Using food as our medicine, what I call food pharmacology, can make a world of difference in healing your adrenals and relieving your symptoms, often in a very short amount of time. The guidelines in this chapter are intended to make it simple and easy. I've also included over forty delicious adrenal-supporting recipes (see "Recipes," page 295) for balancing tonics, smoothies, snacks, and meals, to make the eating plan quick and convenient for you.

Eating a nutrient-rich, blood sugar–balancing, and anti-inflammatory diet is a powerful way to send an abundance of safety messages to your nervous system and is the very first transformation to aid with rebalancing your stress response. But there's even more that we can do, utilizing additional nutritional science strategies, like targeted supplementation and circadian eating, to make your body feel safe.

DIET CAUTIONS

I've created the ATP diet to be the most supportive for restoring an impaired stress response. While the diet can accommodate most food sensitivities, allergies, and diets, some eating styles may contribute to adrenal issues and so are best avoided while you focus on balancing your adrenals.

- **Food sensitivities or allergies:** If you have food sensitivities or allergies to specific foods I say are beneficial, do not eat those foods, even if they are included in the ATP diet. Only do what you know works for you and adapt the recipes as needed.
- **More restrictive diets:** If you follow a more restrictive diet than the one outlined for the program, stick with it. For example, if you are following an autoimmune diet and have eliminated nuts, seeds, and other inflammatory foods as part of that plan, continue to follow those guidelines. Only eat the foods that support your healing.
- **Other specialized diets, such as Whole30, The Zone, and raw foods:** Most eating styles and preferences can be accommodated within the guidelines of the ATP diet, but some recommendations may not be appropriate for those with histamine/oxalate issues. In these cases, I highly recommend working with a practitioner who can help you modify the program to your needs.
- **Fasting:** Fasting can lead to improved insulin sensitivity, an increase in cortisol, and an increase in reverse T3, a hormone that blocks thyroid activity. In healthy individuals, the body perceives these changes as small stressors that help it get into a healing state

known as autophagy, a kind of cellular recycling and resetting in which cells clear out damaged or unnecessary parts and reuse them for repairs or to make new cells. However, those with adrenal issues already have impaired cortisol production, blood sugar imbalances (often presenting as hypoglycemia), an excess of reverse T3, and are undernourished, so fasting can be a *fast way* to increase our stress. I don't recommend fasting until we have addressed these imbalances.

- **Juice fasting:** While we will incorporate green juices into the program, we won't be skipping meals or only drinking juice. Relying solely on stripped-down fruits and vegetables for sustenance, even for just a few days, can add to the protein and other nutrient deficiencies and blood sugar swings contributing to adrenal imbalance and is best avoided for now. Instead, we'll consume juices of fruits and/or vegetables alongside meals with enough fat and/or protein, or we'll blend the juice with healthy fats, such as coconut milk or coconut oil, to counterbalance the blood sugar rush. My recipe Fat Green Juice (page 299) is one of the best ways to get a boost of easy-to-digest vitamins and energy-supporting fats—and beat the mid-morning munchies!

- **Vegan diet/vegetarian diet:** While the vegan and vegetarian diets can be helpful for a variety of conditions, I have not found them to be particularly helpful in healing the adrenals. They can exacerbate blood sugar issues and contribute to deficiencies in important adrenal-supporting nutrients such as the retinol version of vitamin A, B vitamins (especially B_{12}), carnitine, chromium, iron, magnesium, and omega-3s, as well as vitamin D, calcium, iodine, and manganese. Meat-free diets also put us at risk for zinc deficiency and copper excess, which can contribute to adrenal issues, pyroluria, and copper toxicity (some of the recognized causes of adrenal dysfunction). Additionally, vegan/vegetarian sources of protein such as legumes (beans), dairy, grains, and soy may be incompatible with adrenal dysfunction support. Eggs, some seeds, and nuts would be the preferred sources of protein for vegetarians. However, some people, particularly those with inflammatory and/or autoimmune conditions, may be intolerant to those proteins as well, especially in the early stages of starting a healing diet. A diet closer to the hunter-gatherer diet, including nutrient-dense meats, may be more healing during this time.

- **Ketogenic diet:** There are many reported benefits of a high-fat, very low-carb ketogenic diet, including improved energy; blood sugar balance; and reduction of pain, inflammation, migraines, and oxidative stress. It may also contribute to better brain function and mood regulation. Yet many individuals with thyroid and adrenal issues report feeling worse on the keto diet; specifically, they feel more tired. This is often because people with adrenal and thyroid issues have low stomach acid, impaired fatty acid metabolism, and/or deficiencies in fat digestive enzymes, which make it hard for them to extract nutrients from protein and fat. Furthermore, these digestive deficiencies often lead to multiple food sensitivities. With certain adrenal-supporting modifications, such as removing the most common reactive foods (such as dairy) and supplementing with digestive enzymes (see Enzymes in the Advanced Stress Symptom Formulary, page 343) to help break down and absorb proteins and fats, the keto diet can be utilized in this program.

If you would like to get a guide on how to modify the program while eating the keto diet, go to thyroidpharmacist.com/atpbookbonus.

Replenishing with Supplements

Diet and lifestyle are key to recovering from adrenal dysfunction, and you absolutely can do this without supplements. But experience has taught me that supportive supplements can help us heal faster. The chronic stress response results in faster burning of nutrients so we start off with an already nutrient-deficient status. Even when we eat organically grown foods that are higher in nutrients than their conventionally grown, processed counterparts, adrenal dysfunction and autoimmunity both feature digestive issues that impair absorption, leaving us nutrient depleted.

I love using targeted supplements to address the multiple imbalances and deficiencies found in adrenal conditions, such as chronic inflammation, mitochondrial issues, cortisol imbalances, blood sugar swings, and nutrient deficiencies. But taking too many can be overwhelming for our minds, bodies, and pocketbooks. That's why I like to identify supplements that have multiple benefits, to lower your odds of becoming "Pill-bo Baggins." (Why yes, I am a bit of a fangirl of *The Lord of the Rings* and *The Hobbit*.)

One client who came to see me was taking twelve different supplements when she started. Her top complaints were migraines, constipation, insomnia, sensitivity to loud noises, and anxiety. In theory, the protocol she was on was aligned with my approach of supporting the gut, liver, and adrenals that I shared in the Introduction. However, the protocol did not consider her overwhelmed nervous system that was in need of calming before deeper work could be done. I reviewed her list of supplements, had her stop all twelve of them, and recommended just one supplement, magnesium citrate, at bedtime. This is because headaches/migraines, constipation, insomnia, sensitivity to loud noises, and anxiety are all symptoms of a deficiency of magnesium, one of the important nutrients that gets burned up during a stress response. At our follow-up appointment, she reported that her symptoms were gone, including her migraines! She no longer needed to take NSAIDs (nonsteroidal anti-inflammatory drugs), laxatives, or sleep medications, and was able to tolerate her teenager's music (note that I said "tolerate," not "like . . ."—unfortunately there is no supplement or medicine I know of that can make most middle-aged women start loving their teenagers' music!). ☺

I encourage you to consider using a few targeted supplements to address specific symptoms. You might even experience some amazing changes in as little as three days.

ATP SUCCESS STORIES

"The supplements have brought me the biggest change—once I started taking the 'Adrenal Transformation' regimen I started feeling like my old self."

"The supplements and recipes have been very beneficial in lowering inflammation and allowing me to experience more energy, clarity, and inner calmness again."

"Adjusting my diet and adding the supplements have given my body a new strength! I feel more energized and now sleep deeply and for longer. This means I awake refreshed and able to get out of bed with energy that was previously so elusive to me!"

I love that the internet has opened up a whole world of information, and I hope to provide the most helpful and empowering information here, but I also understand that for an already overwhelmed person, more information can be, well, even more overwhelming. Thus while I will share information on various adrenal-supporting supplements for those who wish to do their own experimenting, I will also share my own tried-and-true, streamlined supplement protocol that has helped many people achieve symptom relief.

My protocol includes just six carefully selected supplements to help you restore adrenal balance, listed below in order of importance. Keep reading to discover details about their incredible multitasking healing benefits! In this chapter, we'll cover:

- An adrenal-support supplement containing the ABCs of adrenal balance (adaptogens, B vitamins, and vitamin C) and other minerals.
- Magnesium citrate, often referred to as the "miracle nutrient" because of its multiple healing benefits.
- *Saccharomyces boulardii,* a beneficial yeast-based probiotic that helps resolve gut inflammation.
- Myo-inositol, which supports blood sugar and hormonal balance.

Chapter 5 includes more on:

- An electrolyte blend to maintain optimal fluid balance, reduce inflammation, and balance the circadian rhythm.

- Carnitine, which helps give us energy, promotes blood sugar balance, and supports our mitochondria.

CHOOSING SUPPLEMENTS

Not all supplements are created equal. As a pharmacist, I can tell you that many supplements are ineffective, and some are downright unsafe. The truth is that most supplements do not undergo the same scrutiny and testing that pharmaceutical products do because many of the tests that are required of pharmaceutical companies are "voluntary" for supplement companies. For this reason, most supplement companies do not take the extra steps to test their products to ensure safety and purity.

Evaluating the safety, efficacy, and cost of various treatments was a large part of my training as a pharmacist. I have put my training to good use in overcoming Hashimoto's, evaluating the best supplement brands, and developing my own supplement line, Rootcology. The name "Rootcology" is derived from a blend of my two passions and areas of expertise, root causes and pharmacology: *root*—going after the root cause of disease—and *cology* (as in "pharmacology"), understanding how tiny amounts of substances affect the human body.

Rootcology is dedicated to creating innovative, bioavailable products that are made with the greatest care, and with the highest-quality ingredients available. All of the supplement ingredients have been carefully chosen by yours truly and all Rootcology supplements are:

- Gluten-free
- Dairy-free
- Soy-free
- Pesticide-free
- Toxin-free

- Pharmaceutical grade
- Free from potentially harmful fillers

Furthermore, all Rootcology supplements undergo third-party testing to ensure that the ingredients on the label are safe, effective, and that they match what's actually inside the bottle. I created Rootcology to give you a trusted source of supplements that are safe and effective for people with multiple sensitivities and chronic health conditions.

Throughout this book and in the Advanced Stress Symptom Formulary (page 339), you'll find the supplements I recommend as well as the specific brands to use. I hope this information is helpful on your journey!

I recommended a few of these supplements in the adrenal support protocol in my previous book, *Hashimoto's Protocol*. The additional supplements in my updated ATP reflect what I've since learned about supporting mitochondrial function, electrolyte balance, and building our body's natural resilience. Experience has taught me that this updated program is a more sustainable and effective approach for the majority of people.

Some of the supplements may start working for you in as little as a few days; others might take longer. No matter what, you should start feeling stronger and more energized, and notice your symptoms going away by the end of the program. If you're still feeling symptoms at that point, the last chapter in this book offers guidance on additional interventions to target specific symptoms. Here are some tips on supplementation to keep in mind:

- Generally, you do not need to test your own levels of most nutrients to see if you are deficient. Most have been shown to be safe (with noted precautions) in the research, so my philosophy is to try them and see if they result in improvements. The exceptions are fat-soluble vitamins (A, D, E, and K), copper, and iron, as too much can also cause problems, so I always suggest you check with your practitioner before supplementation. (I don't recommend supplementing with iron, copper, or the fat-soluble vitamins during the four-week program.)

- Speak with your healthcare provider before taking any new supplements, especially if you take prescription medications. Most notably, blood thinners can interact with a lot of adrenal supplements.

- All of the supplements are safe to take with thyroid medications, but note the spacing suggestions for each. I've included this guidance in the Supplement Summary chart in Chapter 8 (page 247), along with recommended doses, brands, and even notes for nursing moms.

Safety of Dietary Changes and Supplements

While the dietary changes and supplements I recommend are generally safe and well tolerated, it's always wise to check with your doctor before changing your diet and starting supplements. Do not stop any medications without the guidance of your doctor. If you are taking thyroid hormones, be sure to retest your levels after starting the diet and supplements, as lifestyle changes can lead to a lower requirement of various medications, including thyroid medications. If you have a history of supplement reactions, please check out the Slow Supplement Introduction Guide for Sensitive Individuals in Appendix 2: How to Modify the Program (page 368) for more guidance. Let's be sure that you are always listening to your body and putting your safety first.

While the ATP meal plan removes the most common inflammatory foods, we are all unique and can develop a sensitivity to any food, even ones that are healing for most people. For example, while coconut milk is full of healthy fats and is a great dairy alternative, some clients have reported that they cannot tolerate coconut. In these cases, I recommend using nut and seed milks instead. If you find that you cannot tolerate some of the most common foods recommended on the ATP diet and in the Recipes, please see the Food Sensitivity Substitution Guide in Appendix 2: How to Modify the Program (page 367).

HOW NOURISHING AND REPLENISHING HELP RESTORE ADRENAL BALANCE

We'll use food as medicine and targeted supplementation to address the most common imbalances caused by being in a prolonged state of chronic stress.

Imbalance	How It Makes You Feel	Why It Happens	How We'll Address It
Blood sugar swings	Hangry, irritable, fatigued, anxious	Dysregulated cortisol also dysregulates insulin, the hormone needed to shuttle blood sugar (glucose) into cells and regulate blood sugar levels.	—Eating a blood sugar–balancing diet, with plenty of good fats and protein. —Adding daily habits to keep blood sugar in check (no skipping breakfast!). —Getting enough myo-inositol, found to help maintain good blood sugar balance, through food and supplementation.
Dysfunctional cortisol production	Tired in the morning and throughout the day, wired at night	Various patterns of cortisol dysfunction, like not enough cortisol during the day/too much cortisol at night, lead to symptoms.	—Circadian nutrition of cortisol-boosting nutrition in the morning and cortisol-lowering approaches in the evenings.

Intestinal permeability (leaky gut)	Stomach pain, digestive distress (diarrhea, constipation, bloating), acid reflux, food sensitivities	Unbalanced levels of cortisol cause inflammation of the digestive tract, leading to gaps in the gut lining and an imbalance of gut flora.	—Removing reactive foods, such as gluten and dairy. —Adding gut-supporting foods. —Supplementing with *Saccharomyces boulardii,* a beneficial yeast that helps clear gut pathogens.
Vitamin A deficiency	Fertility issues, frequent infections, dry skin, night blindness	The active version, retinol, is required to turn cholesterol into pregnenolone, the "mother hormone" needed to make other adrenal hormones.	—Regularly eating foods high in vitamin A. (My recipe for Liver Pâté [page 333] is sure to be a favorite!)
B vitamins deficiencies	Fatigue, low energy, anxiety, insomnia	The B-complex vitamins are needed at every stage of the stress response.	—Regularly eating foods high in B vitamins, such as meat, seafood, poultry, and leafy greens. —Adding an adrenal support supplement with B vitamins.

Vitamin C deficiency	Frequent sickness, slow wound healing, dry skin, easy bruising, joint pain	Vitamin C is needed for the production of cortisol.	—Adding vitamin C–rich foods to our daily diet. —Boosting with an electrolyte supplement blend containing vitamin C. —Adding an adrenal support supplement with vitamin C.
Iron deficiency	Fatigue, weakness, restless legs during sleep, anxiety, insomnia, libido issues	Chronic stress can cause low stomach acid, which significantly reduces iron absorption.	—Supporting stomach acid production with adequate salt intake. —Eating plenty of iron-rich foods, such as red meat, poultry, and pork.
Magnesium deficiency	Muscle cramps, stiffness, insomnia, constipation, anxiety, headaches, sensitivity to loud noises or weakness	Magnesium helps modulate all of the activities of the stress response, including regulating the release of cortisol. Excessive cortisol production depletes magnesium.	—Including magnesium-rich foods in our diet, such as spinach and pumpkin seeds. —Supplementing with magnesium citrate to ensure adequate levels.

Electrolytes (sodium, potassium)	Salt cravings ("I could eat a whole bag of chips!"), dehydration, fatigue, a fast heartbeat, diarrhea or constipation, low blood pressure, low cortisol	As the production of the adrenal hormone aldosterone lessens, more sodium is excreted by the kidneys, leading to frequent urination, electrolyte imbalance, and dehydration.	—Adding sodium, in the form of high-quality sea salt, to foods and beverages. —Consuming high-electrolyte foods, such as bone broth. —Supplementing with an electrolyte blend for complete, balanced support.
Deficiencies in digestive enzymes	Digestive distress (stomach pain, cramps, bloating, gas), low energy (because fat, protein, and other nutrients aren't being properly broken down or absorbed)	Chronic stress downregulates the digestive system and slows the production of digestive enzymes.	—Supplementing with *Saccharomyces boulardii,* a beneficial yeast, found to boost digestive enzymes.
Low stomach acid	Acid reflux, heartburn, indigestion, bloating, trouble digesting meat and protein, food sensitivities	Chronic stress downregulates the digestive system, decreasing blood flow to the stomach, which can decrease the production of stomach acid.	—Adding sodium, in the form of high-quality sea salt, to foods and beverages.

Impaired fatty acid metabolism	Low energy, weakness, irritability	Low cortisol lowers the availability of fat for fuel, and researchers have found that chronic stress stimulates production of a protein that inhibits an enzyme involved in fat metabolism.	—Supplementing with carnitine, which helps convert fat into energy.
Impaired mitochondria function	Low energy, fatigue, exercise intolerance	The high energy demands and inflammation associated with chronic stress "recalibrate" and can even damage the mitochondria so they don't produce energy or adrenal hormones optimally.	—Replenishing with nutrients, such as vitamin A and vitamin C, to reduce damaging oxidative stress and inflammation. —Providing the mitochondria with the nutrients they need to make energy, such as B vitamins, magnesium, and carnitine. —Adding additional energy-supporting compounds such as D-ribose and adaptogens, such as ashwagandha and *Rhodiola rosea*, in an adrenal support blend.

Safety Signal #1: Nutrient Density

My mentor JJ Virgin always says, "Your body is a chemistry lab, not a bank account." In simple words, what we eat matters. Rather than focusing on calories, I encourage you to eat high-quality, nutrient-dense foods, emphasizing fats and proteins, which let the body know that its nutrition needs will be met. Highly processed foods that are full of empty calories send a message that our food supply is scarce, triggering our stress response and survival mode.

Macronutrients

When I was in my first year of pharmacy school, I learned that fat was an essential nutrient. I was shocked! At the time, fat-free diets were a big fad. Unfortunately, many of us have been told that all fat should be avoided, and consequently, we don't eat enough of this essential macronutrient. Fats provide an excellent source of energy, aid the absorption of some vitamins and minerals, build cell membranes, and can help protect us from cardiovascular disease. Fats are also needed to make cholesterol, the precursor for adrenal hormones, and fatty acids that are used up by mitochondria to make energy. Very simply put, a low-fat diet can lead to low levels of the starting materials we need to make our hormones and energy!

After decades of dietary advice proclaiming fats as harmful, both unsaturated fats (found in avocados, olives, nuts, seeds, and certain fish such as salmon and sardines) and types of saturated fats (found mainly in animal sources such as lard and meat and coconut and palm oil) have been found to lower the risk of cardiovascular disease and reduce inflammation.

While cooking, you will want to use coconut or avocado oil, as these are the most stable oils to cook with. It takes higher temperatures for them to smoke and break down, releasing free radicals that can damage cells in the body. Save the olive oil, with a lower smoke point than coconut or avocado oil, for cooking over low heat, drizzling on top of foods, and dressings.

An important concept I want to address is the types of fatty acids present in the fats. The two best known are omega-3 (anti-inflammatory) and omega-6 (pro-inflammatory). Our bodies require both—the right amount of inflammation plays a protective role in our bodies—so omega-6 fats aren't inherently "bad"; rather, the key is to keep them balanced, so we don't end up

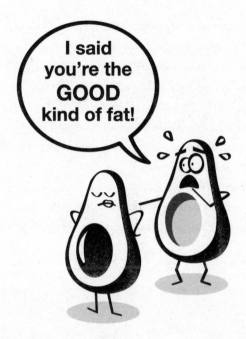

with too much inflammation in the body. The optimal ratio of omega-6 fats to omega-3 fats is 1:1, however people eating most Western diets end up with a ratio closer to 15:1! That means they are getting fifteen times the amount of inflammation needed from the fats they are consuming.

The Balanced Approach to Fats

To restore balance, we will want to limit the intake of fats containing omega-6 acids, as well as dairy-derived omega-3 fats like butter and ghee (due to their propensity to cause food sensitivities, which also increase inflammation) and the recently banned trans fats. Omega-6 acids are most often found in vegetable oils such as canola oil, corn oil, soybean oil, peanut oil, sunflower oil, safflower oil, cottonseed oil, and grapeseed oil, as well as margarine, shortening, nuts, and seeds.

Nuts and seeds highest in omega-6s include peanuts (5320:1 ratio), almonds (2010:1 ratio), and sunflower seeds (311:1 ratio), while walnuts have a more balanced, 4.2:1 ratio.

Conventionally raised animals (vs. the grass-fed, pasture-raised variety) also have higher rates of omega-6s. Trans fats (hydrogenated oils that used to be found in most fried, processed, and packaged foods) have mostly been banned, but manufacturers may still be working through their supplies, and thus they may still be present in some packaged foods.

Due to their anti-inflammatory properties, the omega-3 fatty acids found in seafood can help with balancing cortisol levels and the stress response, so I encourage you to eat lots of low-mercury wild-caught fish such as salmon, sardines, and shellfish.

By eating plenty of omega-3 fats, avoiding processed oils, and swapping conventionally raised meats for grass-fed and pasture-raised versions of the same meats, you'll naturally achieve the right balance.

Healthy Fats	Fats to Avoid
Avocados	Butter*
Avocado oil*	Ghee*
Chia seeds	Meat from conventionally raised
Coconut milk (canned)	animals
Coconut oil	Peanuts
Cod liver oil	Trans fats (hydrogenated oils that
Palm oil (unrefined)	used to be found in most fried,
Duck fat	processed, and packaged foods)
Fish oil	Vegetable oils:
Hazelnuts	corn oil
Hemp seeds	cottonseed oil
MCT oil	canola oil
Olives	safflower oil
Olive oil	soybean oil
Pecans	sunflower oil
Pumpkin seeds	
Salmon	* Butter and ghee are animal-derived
Sardines	saturated fats that can be a great
Shellfish	source of fat, but because so many
Sesame seeds	people are highly sensitive to dairy
Tallow (grass-fed)	proteins, we remove them from the
Walnuts	program to stay on the safe side. *Butter* safe than sorry!

HOW TO INCORPORATE HEALTHY FATS INTO YOUR DAILY ROUTINE

- Use for dressings: 1 tablespoon of extra-virgin olive oil mixed with the freshly squeezed juice of ½ lemon is a great choice!
- Add an avocado to a morning smoothie.
- Top vegetables with a drizzle of extra-virgin olive oil and sprinkle of sea salt.
- For a satisfying snack, drizzle extra-virgin olive oil over slices of avocado and top with a sprinkle of sea salt.
- Add a teaspoon of coconut oil to warm herbal tea (be sure the tea isn't too hot, because you can burn your tongue!). #thingsIlearnedthehardway

Consume Adequate Amounts of High-Quality Protein

Protein is essential for the growth and repair of cells. It is also needed for enzyme and hormone production, detoxification, and to power the fight-or-flight response. Think of protein as the raw fuel to make thyroid hormones, patch up the leaks in your gut, and repair your joints, skin, hair, and nails. And, like fat, it helps to satiate us and keeps us feeling full while balancing our blood sugar.

Yet, many of us are protein deficient as a result of our carb-heavy Western diet or vegan/vegetarian diets or we may not be breaking down and absorbing protein properly. People with adrenal imbalance and/or Hashimoto's are often deficient in the digestive enzymes needed to break down protein into a usable form.

So, how much protein should you have each day? It depends. The average person requires about 1 gram of protein per kilogram of body weight per day (roughly 0.5 grams per pound of body weight). However, people who are over age sixty-five and/or have chronic illness and/or are more active may need up to 1 gram *per pound* of body weight daily. Generally the more active you are, the more protein you need. If you have severe kidney disease and are not on dialysis, you may not be able to tolerate high amounts of protein.

Weight (in pounds)	Protein (in grams)
100	45–100
150	68–150
200	91–200

Keep in mind that a serving of 25 grams of protein can look like:

3 ounces of animal protein, about the size of your palm, OR
4 ounces of fish, about the size of your hand, OR
4 hard-boiled eggs

So, if you have a palm-sized serving of animal protein at each meal, you'll have eaten 75 grams of protein by the end of the day, enough for most people!

Every kind of animal protein is included on the ATP diet so you have an abundance of choice: beef, bison, eggs, lamb, pork, poultry, fish, and shellfish, just to name a few.

While conventionally raised meats contain more inflammatory omega-6 fatty acids than anti-inflammatory omega-3 fatty acids, the reverse is true in naturally raised animals. Look for grass-fed, pasture-raised, wild-caught, and free-range options as well as nitrate- and additive-free deli meats to make sure you are consuming quality proteins that promote healing and repair. Please note that imitation crab often contains gluten and sugar. (Bummer, I know. There goes everyone's favorite fast and easy crab cake recipe!)

It may also be helpful to use protein powders to ensure that you get adequate amounts of (clean) protein. Because the protein is already broken down, it's generally easier to digest than protein from foods. Protein powder also makes it easy to get sufficient protein each day. Just add it to a smoothie! It is important to choose the right kind of protein powder, one that is hypoallergenic and does not include reactive ingredients.

CHOOSING A PROTEIN POWDER

Getting adequate protein throughout the ATP is important, as it helps stabilize blood sugar and provides essential nutrients to fuel the body and support the adrenals.

To boost your protein intake, I recommend including protein powder in your daily routine, but not just any protein powder. Many protein powders on the market contain soy, dairy, grains, and artificial fillers, which can contribute to inflammation and the overall burden on the adrenals. The protein powders that are best tolerated during the adrenal protocol, in my experience, are (from most tolerated to least tolerated):

- **Beef Protein:** Autoimmune friendly and a complete protein, meaning it contains the essential amino acids we need to survive. Hydrolyzed beef protein offers a special advantage, as it is less likely to cause additional food reactions due to the hydrolysis process, which breaks the protein into tiny pieces.
- **Pea Protein:** Vegan, gluten-free, dairy-free, and soy-free and has a mild taste. However, it is not compatible with strict autoimmune protocols. Pea protein can be made from genetically modified peas, so I always recommend choosing only organic pea protein.
- **Hemp Protein:** Vegan, gluten-free, dairy-free, and soy-free, but it has a strong taste that doesn't blend well with some foods, and can be an issue for those with estrogenic concerns. Hemp protein is not compatible with strict autoimmune protocols.

Follow these guidelines to choose a safe protein powder. You may not find a powder that conforms to all of these guidelines, but the more you are able to check off, the better.

- Gluten-free
- Dairy-free (casein, whey, "lactose-free")

- Soy-free (soy isolate, soy protein)
- Grain-free (rice, oats, corn)
- Free of harmful fillers (thickeners and gums, vegetable oils, dextrins, maltodextrins, added fibers)
- Free of artificial sweeteners (aspartame, sucralose, Splenda, saccharin). Stevia is generally well tolerated unless you have a known sensitivity, but it may exacerbate low blood sugar in some cases
- Free of additives, artificial colors, and artificial flavors
- Pesticide-free
- Toxin-free
- GMO-free
- Grass-fed, organic
- Pharmaceutical-grade
- Tested by a third-party lab for safety

Finding it difficult to identify protein powders that are safe, clean, effective, and autoimmune friendly, I spent a great deal of time developing my own. Rootcology protein powders are lab-tested for purity and have been carefully chosen to support healing:

- **AI Paleo Protein (hydrolyzed beef):** Provides 26 grams of protein per serving, and the only ingredient is HydroBEEF, so it's compliant with even the strictest anti-inflammatory protocol. This is a great choice for those who have intolerances or digestive issues, and/or are working on building protocols (such as adrenal recovery).
- **Paleo Protein (hydrolyzed beef):** A vanilla-flavored version of the AI Paleo Protein, which provides 21 grams of protein per serving. This is a great option for those looking for a beef protein source with some flavor (people often compare it to vanilla ice cream!), but please note that it does contain stevia and some light additives.

- **Organic Pea Protein:** An organic, natural pea protein isolate with excellent digestibility and a delicious vanilla flavor. The certified organic North American–grown yellow peas are not genetically modified and are produced with a natural fermentation process that uses no chemical solvents.

Additional clean proteins I recommend are:

- Designs for Health PurePaleo Unflavored (beef protein)
- Designs for Health PurePaleo Vanilla (beef protein)
- Designs for Health Organic PurePea Vanilla
- NOW Foods Pea Protein
- Manitoba Harvest Hemp Yeah! Max Protein Unsweetened Hemp Protein Powder

Adaptogens

We can build the body's resilience to stress and improve nutrient extraction by promoting a healthy stress response (where the body returns to "rest and digest" mode after experiencing stress) with adaptogenic herbs. These are the "A" of the ABCs for balancing the adrenals I mentioned in Chapter 1.

Adaptogenic herbs comprise many natural herb products that help the body deal with stressors. In the 1940s, pharmacologist Nikolai Lazarev first defined the concept of adaptogens: a substance that can raise the body's resilience to various types of stress, including physical and emotional stress.

In order to be considered an adaptogen, an herb must possess several qualities. First, it must be nontoxic at normal doses. Second, the herb should help the entire body cope with stress. Third, it should help the body return to balance regardless of how the stress is currently affecting the person's function. In other words, an adaptogenic herb needs to be able to both tone down overactive systems (normalize too much cortisol production) and boost underactive systems (increase cortisol production) in the body.

I find that using adaptogens helps keep me balanced, especially during my own peak periods of stress (did someone say "holidays" or "book deadline"?) and I have joked in the past that adaptogens make all the people in my life much easier to tolerate. I did stop them during pregnancy, and besides my little one's arrival and sleeping on my belly again, getting back on adaptogens was one of the things I looked forward to the most. Adaptogenic herbs include:

- **American ginseng:** One of my favorites because of its many benefits! In research, it has been found to have anti-inflammatory, anti-fatigue, and antiaging effects. Its ginsenoside content is thought to play a role in these benefits, and animal experiments have shown that ginsenosides have the ability to improve working memory (bye-bye, brain fog!).
- **Ashwagandha:** Another favorite and rightly popular herb found to have many anti-stress properties. In addition to reducing anxiety and improving one's overall mood, ashwagandha has been shown to be calming, anti-inflammatory, pain-relieving, and beneficial for libido and normalizing thyroid hormone levels. Ashwagandha also contains a significant amount of iron, a huge plus, as iron deficiency is common in those with adrenal imbalance. (Ashwagandha should be avoided by people with nightshade sensitivity.)
- **Astragalus:** This adaptogen supports improved immune function and is often used to decrease fatigue.
- **Dang shen:** Research has found that Dang shen has many bioactive properties, and I like recommending it for supporting the immune system and gastrointestinal function.
- **Eleuthero (Siberian ginseng):** My go-to for those who work too hard and play too hard! It has been shown to boost mitochondrial activity, increase endurance and stamina, and improve recovery after exercise.
- **Holy basil (tulsi):** Its many anti-inflammatory, mood-stabilizing, and antianxiety benefits have been well documented. It optimizes cortisol

levels when altered by stress and lowers blood sugar in type 2 diabetes. It's also been shown to increase blood circulation to the brain, helping improve memory and reduce brain fog. I love drinking tulsi tea to support my overall stress levels.

- **Jiaogulan:** In addition to helping regulate the stress response, studies suggest that jiaogulan may help control blood sugar levels. Drinking jiaogulan tea has been shown to reduce fasting blood sugar levels and improve insulin sensitivity in people with diabetes.

- **Licorice:** Licorice helps increase energy levels by preventing the breakdown of cortisol, and thereby lessening the demand on the adrenals to produce more of it. It works well for morning fatigue seen in advanced stages of adrenal dysfunction (low cortisol), and it's best when taken in the morning. Licorice has also been found to lower inflammation and has antiviral and gut-healing properties. (Licorice should be avoided by those who have high blood pressure and/or high cortisol levels.)

- **Maca (Peruvian ginseng):** I have found that it helps my clients with their energy levels and overall mood, as well as symptoms of hormone imbalance (brain fog, memory, metabolism, hot flashes). Maca has been shown to reduce anxiety and depression, and clinical trials found that it may also improve sexual desire and libido.

- **Reishi mushroom:** A medicinal mushroom with excellent immune-boosting properties (in particular for upper respiratory viral infections), reishi can balance mood swings caused by excess androsterone conversion. This is a great choice for when you are looking for more "chill" in your life. I like to drink reishi tea during the day and in the evenings for more restful sleep.

- **Rhodiola rosea:** An energy-boosting powerhouse! Studies have shown it helps relieve fatigue; promote a positive mood; and improve sleep, brain function, and symptoms of burnout. In one study, participants with chronic fatigue symptoms who received 400 mg of rhodiola every day for eight weeks experienced significant improvements in fatigue, mood, concentration, and overall quality of life. Improvements were observed after only one week and continued throughout the study. In animal studies, rhodiola has been found to enhance mitochondrial function, significantly increasing exercise capacity and reducing the oxidative stress damage to muscles. The combination of anti-stress effects and increased available energy is why I love rhodiola for adrenal support.

- **Schisandra:** Schisandra has been shown to help in states of exhaustion, to increase alertness, improve the ability to learn and memorize, and improve mental performance and overall concentration. It's also been found to be beneficial as a sleep aid.

- **Shatavari:** The word "Shatavari" itself means "woman of a hundred husbands." I'm not sure if the interpretation is focused on the stress of having a hundred husbands or the libido requirement, but this herb has powerful hormone-balancing effects for women, which include being a galactagogue to aid milk production, balancing PCOS, supporting libido and fertility, as well as having antidepressant and aphrodisiac properties.

- **Suma:** Suma is used for its anti-fatigue, anti-inflammatory, anti-stress, and immune supportive properties. It has been found to be effective in relieving pain.

SUPPLEMENT SPOTLIGHT #1: ADRENAL SUPPORT BLEND

You can get adaptogens as stand-alone products depending on your unique circumstances. For convenience, improved efficacy through synergy, and so that you don't have to pop twenty different pills a day, I usually recommend taking an adrenal support blend that contains a mix of synergistic adaptogens (the A's) as well as the common vitamins that become depleted due to chronic stress (the B's and C).

I created Rootcology Adrenal Support Blend to include five carefully chosen, synergistic adaptogens: ashwagandha, American ginseng, eleuthero, licorice, and rhodiola rosea due to their unique, multipurpose properties. When used together, they address most of the causes of adrenal symptoms: low cortisol levels (rhodiola, licorice), blood sugar metabolism, mitochondrial function (rhodiola, eleuthero), viral infections (licorice), gut inflammation (licorice), low T3 levels (ashwagandha), and low iron levels (ashwagandha).

As my clients' chief complaint is usually fatigue, I chose to include adaptogens that are helpful with energy, endurance, and performance, including licorice, eleuthero, and American ginseng. Additionally, Rootcology Adrenal Support contains the amino acid N-acetyl L-tyrosine, a precursor to the mood- and focus-boosting dopamine, adrenaline, and thyroxine (T4), a main thyroid hormone, for additional brain fog, focus, thyroid, and energy support. The blend also contains the B vitamins and vitamin C, two of the most commonly depleted nutrients in adrenal dysfunction (more about that below).

Please note that this blend has been specially formulated with licorice, which helps us increase our cortisol levels; thus it's best taken in the morning when we want our cortisol to be higher. This blend is excellent for people with low cortisol or experiencing the cortisol roller coaster. Additionally, Rootcology Adrenal Support should be avoided in people with high blood pressure and/or high cortisol levels. A better product for those with high blood pressure and/or high cortisol levels is the Daily Stress Formula by Pure Encapsulations.

If you only take one supplement as part of the ATP, I recommend taking an adrenal support blend that contains the ABCs. Program participants are encouraged to start an adrenal support blend during the first or second week. After about three days or so at the right dose, you should start seeing some improvements in your energy levels and ability to handle whatever curveballs the day throws at you! If needed, I also encourage you to use additional, complementary adaptogens as teas. Some favorites are Maca Latte, also known as "hello, libido" (page 300), tulsi tea for day-to-day balancing of the stress response (delicious on its own, or as the Tulsi Tea Latte on page 302), and reishi (my favorite blend is the hot cocoa blend by Four Sigmatic), for a relaxing evening treat to help with winding down.

Adrenal support blends should be taken with caution, and it's important to note that results may vary. Consult your healthcare practitioner before use if you are pregnant or lactating or if you have hypertension or diabetes or have had kidney or liver disorders. Discontinue use and consult your healthcare practitioner if you experience sleeplessness, headache, bleeding, or heart palpitations.

Some adrenal support blends on the market may contain ingredients that haven't sat well with some of my clients or may require testing to be used safely. These include:

- Glandular adrenal extracts, which are made from the adrenal glands of animals. Whole-gland adrenal extracts contain norepinephrine and epinephrine, which can cause anxiety, palpitations, and panic attacks due to a shock of adrenaline. Adrenal extracts can cause HPA axis suppression and atrophy, meaning that they can turn off the production of the body's own steroid (adrenal) hormones.
- Cortisol-lowering ingredients that include magnolia bark or high doses of phosphatidylserine need to be avoided in those with cortisol that's already low.
- Pregnenolone, DHEA, and 7-Keto DHEA are hormones that can be unsafe when used by the wrong person at the wrong times (see more on page 8).
- If you have high blood pressure, you will want to avoid licorice-containing blends, like Rootcology Adrenal Support.
- If you have a nightshade sensitivity, avoid ashwagandha-containing blends, including Rootcology Adrenal Support.
- While some adaptogens are safe for nursing moms and their babies, and may promote milk supply, I don't recommend adrenal support

blends for nursing moms due to potentially problematic ingredients. Some ginsengs and B$_6$ in excess of 50 mg can lower prolactin levels, while eleutherococcus can lead to excess bleeding. Rather, I recommend utilizing holy basil (tulsi), shatavari, reishi, and/or rhodiola, starting with one herb at a time. These four are the gentlest of the adaptogens and most often used in lactation. Holy basil and shatavari may promote milk supply, so be sure to discuss with your lactation consultant. You may also wish to add a B-complex vitamin that has under 50 mg of vitamin B$_6$ to the mix or use individual B vitamins. Vitamin C supplements are generally safe for nursing moms and may help as well.

Nutrients

Replenishing the nutrients that become depleted in fight-or-flight mode is essential to restoring adrenal balance and overall health. In addition to eating plenty of good fats and adequate protein, we'll aim to incorporate foods high in the most important nutrients required for adrenal health.

- Vitamin A
- B vitamins
- Vitamin C
- Iron
- Magnesium
- Electrolytes, such as sodium (covered in "Electrolytes" [page 152]).

Vitamin A

This essential nutrient does so much more than keep our eyesight sharp! Retinol, the active version of vitamin A, is required to turn cholesterol into pregnenolone, the "mother hormone" needed to make other adrenal hormones, and it plays an important role in skin protection, mitochondrial health, and reproductive health. It regulates the immune system response so it doesn't become overactive—as seen in autoimmune diseases—and strengthens its ability to fight infections and clear pathogens. Vitamin A also helps heal the gut by supporting the intestinal lining.

Our bodies don't make vitamin A, so we need it from our diet. Animal foods, such as liver, egg yolks, and seafood, contain the most easily absorbed and bioavailable version (retinol). Beef liver is the richest source of retinol, and while I know liver may not be to everyone's taste, I encourage you to try it—seasoning can make all the difference (see the Liver Pâté recipe on page 333).

But what about carrots? Your mom wasn't wrong when she said bright orange and yellow vegetables give us better vision, but she may not have known that they don't contain vitamin A in a form the body can readily use. Orange and yellow vegetables (yellow peppers, sweet potatoes, golden beets) and fruits (oranges, lemons) contain beta-carotene, which can convert to retinol. For some people, this just means that plant foods are a less efficient way to get vitamin A and we need to eat more of them to get enough each day—nothing wrong with that! Studies suggest that consuming beta-carotene-rich plants with some fat, like drizzling extra-virgin olive oil over a spinach salad, can also improve absorption.

However, for others like me (estimates suggest about 45 percent of the population), a genetic variation on the BCMO1 gene significantly impairs the body's ability to convert beta-carotene into retinol, making it very difficult to get enough vitamin A from plant foods alone. Individuals with this variation need to prioritize animal sources.

If you're not sure about your genes, the best way to make sure you're getting enough vitamin A is to eat a variety of foods. I don't recommend supplementation (unless under the supervision of your healthcare provider) because excess vitamin A is stored in your body and too much can lead to toxicity. Instead, aim to regularly eat foods high in vitamin A (or its precursors), including:

Beef liver, pan fried, 3 ounces: 6,582 mcg
Sweet potato, baked in skin, one whole: 1,403 mcg
Spinach, raw, 1 cup: 2,813 IU
Carrots, raw, ½ cup: 459 mcg

Orange juice, raw, 1 cup: 496 IU

Pepper, sweet yellow, raw, one large: 372 IU

Broccoli, raw, ½ cup: 274 IU

Egg, poached, one large: 242 IU

Salmon, sockeye, cooked, 3 ounces: 59 mcg

Lemon juice, raw, 1 ounce: 5.6 IU

How to incorporate more vitamin A–rich foods into your diet:

- Have beef liver for your lunch or dinner one to two times each week. Try my Liver Pâté recipe (page 333). Use strong seasonings to make it tastier. I like turmeric for its flavor and anti-inflammatory kick! You can also sneak liver into a favorite lunch or dinner dish like meatballs by grinding it up in a food processor and mixing it with the rest of the ground beef or turkey in the recipe. Try it with my Butternut Spaghetti & Turkey Meatballs (page 311).
- Add spinach, carrots, and lemon juice to your morning smoothie.
- Add chopped red or yellow peppers to a salad.

B vitamins

There are eight nutrients that collectively make up the B complex: B_1 (thiamine), B_2 (riboflavin), B_3 (niacin), B_5 (pantothenic acid), B_6 (pyridoxine), B_7 (biotin), B_9 (folate), and B_{12} (cobalamin). These play an important role in cell metabolism, thyroid function, and adrenal function. All of them are necessary throughout every step of the stress response, from supporting energy production (the stress response requires a lot of energy!) to adrenal hormone production. B vitamins become depleted during high cortisol production, and deficiencies in pantothenic acid (B_5) and biotin (B_7) in particular have been linked to decreased adrenal function in animals and humans.

Vegans and vegetarians are at the greatest risk of vitamin B_{12} deficiency because it must be consumed (the body can't synthesize it) and it is only found in animal foods, such as meat and dairy products, but people with autoimmune and gut issues also have higher rates of vitamin B_{12} deficiency.

Foods high in one or more B vitamins include meat, seafood, poultry, leafy greens, and sunflower seeds (one of the best plant sources of pantothenic acid).

How to incorporate more B vitamins into your diet:
- Add leafy greens to a morning smoothie.
- Include a B vitamin–rich protein for lunch and dinner each day.
- Add sunflower seeds to a salad.

A supplement containing a variety of B vitamins will be helpful for most people with adrenal imbalance, especially those experiencing low energy and fatigue. You can take B vitamins on an individual basis, as a combination B vitamin supplement, often formulated as B-complex blends (B-Complex by Pure Encapsulations is an excellent product), or as part of an adrenal support blend of the ABCs.

I created Rootcology Adrenal Support to use a combination of B vitamins, along with adaptogens, a small dose of vitamin C, and L-Tyrosine to support the adrenals, in one convenient formula. Other adrenal support blends I like that include B vitamins are Designs for Health Adrenotone and Pure Encapsulations Daily Stress Formula.

B vitamins are water-soluble, so they do not build up in the body; the risk for toxicity is almost nonexistent, with the exception of vitamin B_6, which can cause neurological issues at doses above 300 mg per day. In people with severe deficiencies, additional doses of B vitamins may be needed beyond what's in an adrenal support blend or a B-complex supplement, such as riboflavin, thiamine, biotin, B_6, folate (as methylfolate, the most bioavailable version), or B_{12}. A mix of Bs is a great place to start, and if needed, recommendations for additional B vitamins can be found in the Nutrient Guide of the Advanced Stress Symptom Formulary (page 352), to help you select the most beneficial types and dosing.

Vitamin C
The adrenal glands rely on vitamin C to function and manufacture cortisol, which makes it essential for adrenal healing and restoring balance to the HPA axis. Because it gets burned up quickly due to chronic stress, proper

replenishment is essential. Vitamin C also helps support the immune system, collagen production, and the eradication of Epstein-Barr virus infections, along with many other potential viruses. A powerful antioxidant, vitamin C also scavenges free radicals, which are unstable oxygen atoms that damage other cells or parts of cells, such as the mitochondria.

Choosing vitamin C–rich recipes, such as the Adrenal Kick Start (page 297), Deli Wraps/Bell Pepper Sandwich (page 331), and Salmon & Brussels Sprout Salad (page 310), and adding other foods high in vitamin C to your daily diet will feed and support your adrenals.

Foods high in vitamin C include:
Acerola cherries, raw, ½ cup: 822 mg
Sweet yellow peppers, raw, ½ cup: 137 mg
Mustard spinach, raw, 1 cup: 195 mg
Kale, raw, 1 cup: 80 mg
Kiwi, one unit: 71 mg
Broccoli, raw or steamed, ½ cup: 40.5 mg
Brussels sprouts, raw, ½ cup: 37.5 mg
Strawberries, raw, 1 cup: 89 mg
Orange, raw, one medium: 70 mg

How to incorporate vitamin C–rich foods into your daily routine:
- Add fruits or greens to your smoothie.
- Rotate between broccoli, Brussels sprouts, and other greens with lunch and dinner.
- For a snack, have a piece of fruit and some fat (like a kiwi with almonds).

My favorite way to boost vitamin C is through an electrolyte blend powder, such as Rootcology's Electrolyte Blend (see Supplement Spotlight #5). This powder contains 1,734 mg of vitamin C, along with other vital nutrients and minerals to support hydration. Designs for Health's Electrolyte Synergy is another great vitamin C–containing blend. Some people may also benefit from a stand-alone vitamin C supplement, such as NOW Foods

Chewable C-500. I recommend a total daily intake of 500 to 3,000 mg of vitamin C, as tolerated.

Iron

Over the years I've seen so many clients become more energized and emotionally balanced, experience less brain fog, and improve their sleep after addressing low iron levels.

Women who are pregnant or recently postpartum are at high risk for iron deficiency. Low iron levels are also found in up to 50 percent of women of childbearing age (heavy menses due to hypothyroidism or progesterone deficiency can be one cause here). The rates are higher in vegans, vegetarians, and individuals with gut and thyroid conditions. Additionally, low iron levels are a sign that the body is under stress and can lead to an increased production of reverse T3.

On the ATP diet, we'll start by using food as medicine to maintain proper iron levels. Iron is present in both heme and non-heme versions in different foods. The heme version is the better-absorbed version and is found primarily in animal products. The highest levels of iron are found in organ meats (more liver . . . sorry!). Beef, turkey, and chicken are the next best choices. Non-heme iron is found in plant foods such as nuts, beans, and spinach and is not usually absorbed as well, which is why the recommended daily allowance of iron is almost double for people who eat a plant-based diet compared to that of meat eaters. Eating vitamin C–rich foods, such as broccoli, with non-heme sources of iron can dramatically increase iron absorption.

Foods high in iron include:
   Beef liver, cooked, 1 slice: 5.0 mg
   Beef, ground, 3 ounces: 2.2 mg
   Turkey, light meat, cooked, 1 cup: 1.9 mg
   Chicken breast, cooked, 1 cup: 1.5 mg
   Cashews, raw, 1 ounce: 1.9 mg
   Spinach, raw, 1 cup: 0.8 mg

How to incorporate iron-rich foods into your diet:

- Eat cooked liver twice per week. If you're not a fan of liver (yet!), try adding seasonings to improve the taste or grind the liver and add to other meat dishes to "hide" it.
- Eat beef for lunch or dinner a few times per week.
- On other days, have turkey or chicken as your protein with lunch or dinner.

IS DIETARY IRON ENOUGH?

In cases where food isn't enough to maintain adequate iron levels, or if you just can't look at liver without wanting to cry, supplements may help. We won't be utilizing iron supplements in the four-week program because iron is a nutrient that requires testing before supplementing and retesting your levels within one to three months, to ensure that you are supplementing enough—but not too much, as elevated iron levels can become toxic. That said, if you have any residual symptoms after the four-week program, I recommend testing your iron levels, specifically your ferritin level. Iron deficiency (commonly seen in children and women of child-bearing age) and iron toxicity (more often seen in men and postmenopausal women and those with certain genetic conditions) can both contribute to adrenal stress symptoms. Please refer to the Nutrient Guide in the Advanced Stress Symptom Formulary (page 352) for guidance on testing and recommended supplementation.

Magnesium

Magnesium is necessary for more than three hundred biochemical reactions in the body, supporting everything from the immune system to nerve and muscle function and blood glucose and energy levels. The cells in your adrenal glands need magnesium to operate, but it can become depleted with excessive cortisol production. Magnesium is also fundamental to the stress response, as it helps regulate the secretion of cortisol and supports healthy levels of DHEA, the youth hormone. So while the body requires magnesium for a healthy stress response, it can exhaust its supply when the HPA axis is in overdrive. Even though magnesium is so important, a significant number of people are deficient in it (an estimated 50 percent of the U.S. population).

While it may be challenging to get enough magnesium from foods, foods high in magnesium include:

Pumpkin seeds, 1 ounce: 168 mg
Almonds, 1 ounce: 80 mg
Spinach, boiled, ½ cup: 78 mg
Cashews, 1 ounce: 7 mg
Avocado, 1 cup: 44 mg
Chicken breast, roasted, 3 ounces: 22 mg
Beef, lean, ground, 3 ounces: 20 mg
Broccoli, cooked, ½ cup: 10 mg

How to incorporate magnesium-rich foods into your daily routine:
- Add some seeds or nuts to salads.
- Add ½ cup of cooked spinach to your lunch or dinner. I like adding it to soup!
- For a satisfying snack, smash an avocado with lime juice, salt, and pepper and a drizzle of extra-virgin olive oil (all to taste). Dig in with your favorite veggies.

SUPPLEMENT SPOTLIGHT #2: MAGNESIUM

Because magnesium is often difficult to obtain from foods and is depleted by stress, deficiency is very, very common, especially in those with stress response symptoms. That is why I often recommend supplementation.

Research supports the benefits my clients have experienced after taking a bedtime magnesium supplement, including increased calm, better sleep, more energy, and relief from constipation, menstrual and muscle cramps, migraines, and anxiety. Magnesium has also been shown to normalize the thyroid's appearance on an ultrasound in some people with Hashimoto's, if taken for at least eight months, and may also help thyroid and breast nodules.

Oral magnesium supplements are available in different forms. I recommend taking magnesium citrate because it tends to be more calming and sleep-promoting than magnesium glycinate, though it does have more stool-softening properties. Also, for some people glycinate can worsen anxiety.

Rootcology Magnesium Citrate Powder provides 300 mg of magnesium in each one-teaspoon serving, in a convenient powder form, so that dosing can be easily adjusted to individual needs. I also like Designs for Health's MagCitrate Powder, as well as Pure Encapsulations Magnesium (citrate for most, or glycinate for those prone to loose stools). The usual starting dose ranges for magnesium are magnesium citrate at 400 mg, and magnesium glycinate at 100 mg, at bedtime. That said, please note that the dosages depend on the formulation of magnesium, so always check the label.

Getting sufficient magnesium can lead to great improvements in many symptoms. Program participants have shared how much magnesium has helped them get rid of their muscle aches, sleep issues/fatigue, IBS issues, headaches, and cramps, as well as improving libido:

> "The magnesium citrate is a life changer. No trouble anymore getting to sleep and I'm sure I'm getting better sleep since being on it."
>
> "Magnesium got rid of the muscle aches almost immediately!"
>
> "I take magnesium bisglycinate and citrate and that has helped me immensely. No more IBS issues, headaches, and cramps."

Additional Tips for Sending Your Body Nutrient Density Safety Signals

- **Choose smoothies:** Smoothies are a great-tasting, nutrient-packed way to start your day without digestive stress. Chopping up the ingredients in a blender renders the food easier to digest and the nutrients easier to absorb. Adding one serving of protein powder to your morning smoothie makes sure you're getting adequate amounts of protein each day while helping to stabilize your blood sugar and reduce inflammation. (See Choosing a Protein Powder on page 113.)

  Many of my clients have reported seeing a marked difference in their energy levels after adding my smoothies to their routine—without the need for caffeine! In fact, a lot of people never go back to caffeine because they feel so much better! Check out my favorite: the Root Cause Green Smoothie (page 304), combining a program-compliant protein powder, healthy fats (coconut milk, avocado), and nutrient-rich veggies!

- **Eat until we're full and satisfied:** There's no calorie counting or restrictions on the ATP diet! Depriving our bodies of food sends a message that we are in a famine and therefore not safe (this is why I do not recommend fasting as part of this program). On the other hand, eating a lot of the right kinds of foods lets our bodies and brains know that it has enough of what it needs to keep us going—in other words, the body feels safe, so eating like this is an important safety signal. We want our bodies to know that there is plenty of food and stay in a rest, digest, and healing mode.

- **Consume six to eight servings of non-starchy nutrient-rich vegetables:** If you've ever heard the term "eat the rainbow," that's exactly my recommendation to help you get a variety of nutrients! Non-starchy vegetables—think leafy greens (spinach, collards, Swiss chard), leeks, cucumbers, broccoli, cauliflower, Brussels sprouts, and cabbage—are packed with nutrients and can also help maintain stable blood sugar levels.

THYROID TIP: THE TRUTH ABOUT CRUCIFEROUS VEGETABLES AND HASHIMOTO'S

There's a myth that those with Hashimoto's should avoid cruciferous vegetables because they contain glucosinolate, a substance that, when consumed in large quantities, can prevent the thyroid from uptaking iodine. This could be an issue for someone who has iodine deficiency–induced hypothyroidism, but most people with Hashimoto's do not have an iodine deficiency, and most cruciferous vegetables don't have enough glucosinolates to induce one. In my experience, most cruciferous vegetables are well tolerated by people with Hashimoto's and provide important health benefits, including helping the body detoxify.

- **Add nutrient-dense superfoods:** If you're looking for a way to incorporate more nutrients into your diet, consider the following boosters! Many of them are not just nutritious but also delicious and can be added to drinks, smoothies, salads, and other foods. There are also a couple that taste, let's just say "medicinal." ☺ They are best used as "wellness shots."

Product	Booster For	Where to Use	How Much
Black cumin seed spice	Gut health, blood sugar balance	As spice in topping on salads; as oil as a wellness shot	1 tablespoon (2 grams) per day
Blueberries	myo-inositol, blood sugar balance, thyroid hormone support	In smoothies, salads, snacks (when combined with protein/fat)	½ to 1 cup per day
Bone broth (recipe on page 305)	Gut health	In soups and stews, as a drink	½ to 4 cups a day
Camu camu powder	Vitamin C	In smoothies, drinks	¼ to ½ teaspoon per day

Product	Booster For	Where to Use	How Much
Chia seeds	Healthy fats	In smoothies, salads	1 to 2 tablespoons per day
Cinnamon	Blood sugar balance	In drinks, lattes, and fruit	A pinch to ½ teaspoon per day
Coconut oil	Healthy fats, blood sugar balance	In frying, cooking vegetables; add to warm beverages, juices to support blood sugar balance	½ teaspoon-plus per day
Coconut milk	Boost fat, antiviral	In smoothies, soups, dressings	¼ cup-plus per day
Coconut yogurt	Gut microbiome balance	In smoothies, dressings, as a snack	Start with ½ to 2 teaspoonfuls
Cod liver oil	Lower inflammation	In salads, seafood	½ to 1 teaspoonful daily
Fermented coconut water	Gut microbiome balance	As a "wellness shot" or beverage mixer	Start with ½ ounce daily; increase over time
Fermented vegetables	Gut microbiome balance	As side dishes, on top of salad	Start with ½ teaspoon daily; work your way up
Liver	Iron, vitamin A	In recipes (Liver Pâté, page 333); in meatballs or meat sauce	4 ounces per week
Maca powder	Hormone balance, libido	In Maca Latte (page 300), smoothies, coconut yogurt topping	1 to 3 teaspoons
Pumpkin pie spice	Blood sugar balance, reduce inflammation	In lattes, smoothies, fruit	A pinch-plus daily
Pumpkin seeds	Boost magnesium, balance blood sugar	In salads and in snacks	A tablespoon or more
Sea salt	Balance blood pressure, support cortisol	On everything; in Sole (page 301)	A pinch-plus daily
Turmeric spice	Reduce inflammation	In a "wellness shot" in drinks, cooking in foods	A pinch-plus daily

Safety Signal #2: Lowered Inflammation

There are so many reasons why we may have inflammation in our bodies. Some reasons are obvious; others are hidden and it may take some detective work to find them. Because our body is so interconnected and because the stress response weakens our gut, no matter the original reason for the inflammation, supporting the gut will send a powerful message of safety and will help with addressing stress response symptoms.

Reduce Gut Inflammation

Poor gut health can be a major source of chronic inflammation, a top four stressor underlying adrenal imbalance and autoimmune thyroid conditions. We will focus on reducing inflammation in the digestive system by removing the top inflammatory foods, adding gut-supporting foods, and using beneficial yeast called *Saccharomyces boulardii,* which can help with reducing the gut's reactivity to foods, establishing a healthy gut flora, and displacing inflammation-inducing gut pathogens.

Remove Reactive Foods

Certain foods can trigger an autoimmune response in the body and lead to widespread inflammation. These dietary irritants can cause toxic reactions in the body—we call these food sensitivities. Food sensitivities are different from allergies in that they are produced by the IgG and IgA branch of the immune system, whereas food allergies are mediated by the IgE branch of the immune system.

Food sensitivities and food allergies also differ in the reactions they produce in the body. A food sensitivity will produce symptoms such as irritable bowel syndrome, headaches, dizziness, brain fog, joint pain, acid reflux, anxiety, skin breakouts, itchiness, postnasal drip, congestion, heart palpitations, fatigue, and insomnia, which may take up to four days to appear, while an allergic reaction is likely to appear immediately and be much more severe, often involving hives, itching, or swelling of the throat and mouth and difficulty breathing.

By removing the most common reactive foods in the Western diet as well as other foods that can stress the body and interfere with healing, we can reduce inflammation, support a healthy gut, and promote adrenal balance.

Removing reactive foods from the diet can result in a noticeable improvement in symptoms in a matter of days, though complete healing may take several weeks or months. The majority of my clients report feeling significantly better after removing the following foods from their diet.

Gluten
Many people, especially those with blood sugar issues and autoimmune disease, are sensitive to gluten, a protein found in grains such as barley, rye, wheat, and packaged foods. Gluten can lead to an inflammatory gut response that can last from minutes to weeks per ingestion, depending on the spectrum of sensitivity. It is also possible that you have celiac disease, in which case you could experience a more severe form of these reactions and have them immediately after eating a gluten-containing food.

Gluten-free grains
For this program, we remove gluten and *all* grains, including grains that are considered gluten-free, to ensure that any substances that might inflame the gut lining are removed, and to support blood sugar balance. Even though gluten-free grains don't contain gluten, they can cross-react with gluten and can significantly spike our blood sugar. Grains to avoid include barley, buckwheat, bulgur, corn, durum, farro, kamut, maize, quinoa, oats, rice, rye, semolina, spelt triticale, and wheat.

Dairy
There are various reasons the body may respond to dairy with inflammation, including the quality of dairy, lactose intolerance, or sensitivity to the casein and whey proteins found in dairy products. For the program we will be eliminating all sources of cow, goat, and sheep dairy, including milk, cheese, cream, yogurt, ice cream, butter, ghee, and certain protein powders.

Soy
Soy is a type of legume used to make many meat- and dairy-free foods. It's also frequently used in processed foods to bind ingredients together or add texture. Soy protein sensitivity is very common, and so we will steer clear of edamame, soy milk, tofu, tempeh, miso, soy sauce, and processed

foods and supplements, which often contain soy-based ingredients. This includes gluten-free, vegan, and vegetarian products, which can contain soy lecithin, bean curd, hydrolyzed soy protein, and/or hydrolyzed vegetable protein.

Other legumes, except green beans and pea protein

Legumes contain phytates that bind to nutrients and lead to poor zinc absorption. Phytates are linked to increased gut permeability and infections. Legumes to avoid include beans (black beans, soybeans, fava beans, garbanzo beans or chickpeas, kidney beans, lima beans), lentils, and peanuts. Green beans and pea protein are generally more well tolerated and thus included on the four-week diet.

Sugar

Not only does sugar contribute to blood sugar swings and inflammation, it can exacerbate an imbalanced gut microbiome. Avoid table sugar (sucrose) and processed foods that contain sugar or high-fructose corn syrup. Sugar lurks in many places, including grains, especially gluten-free grains and treats, alcohol, fruit juice, fruit, prepackaged food, and conventional meats.

We want to minimize sweeteners, but if having them will make it easier to adhere to the diet, stevia, maple syrup, monk fruit, and honey are the best sugar substitutes. (Please use them in moderation.)

Seaweed

Because having adrenal issues puts us at risk for autoimmune conditions, including Hashimoto's, we are avoiding seaweed due to its propensity to modulate the immune system and high iodine content, a known trigger for Hashimoto's in those genetically predisposed to it. I recommend eliminating all types of seaweed: nori, kombu, kelp, and wakame.

Spicy peppers

Capsaicin, the ingredient in peppers that makes them spicy, can cause leaky gut, so peppers with this compound are to be avoided. Capsaicin-containing spicy peppers include chili peppers, Thai peppers, red chili flakes, and cayenne pepper. Black pepper (*Piper nigrum*) gets its "spice" from piperine, not capsaicin, so it won't produce the same inflammatory reaction and can be used safely. Bell peppers are also well tolerated by most.

Alcohol

Alcohol causes blood sugar imbalances, leaky gut, and an overgrowth of bacteria in the small intestine, as well as a buildup of inflammatory toxins like ammonia in the body. We will avoid all types of alcohol during the four-week program, and yes, this includes wine, although many of us would like to think it has health benefits (the jury is of course still out, but for the purposes of this program, we will not be drinking rosé all day—sorry!).

SHOPPING FOR QUALITY INGREDIENTS

If you're unsure about a particular type of food, think about whether ancient humans would have been eating it (I call this the "caveperson test").

We also need to be aware that conventionally grown crops have varying degrees of pesticide residue, such as glyphosate, a popular herbicide and mitochondrial toxin.

Conventionally grown produce also tends to have a lower nutrient content, in part because it is grown in repeatedly used, nutrient-depleted soil. This is one of the reasons we often need to supplement, even when eating a nutritious diet, and why I encourage you to purchase organic foods whenever possible. Studies have shown that organic fruits and vegetables have lower levels of pesticide residue and higher levels of antioxidants, which have anti-inflammatory benefits.

Meats: Look for local, organic, grass-fed, and/or wild-caught meat when possible. The shorter the distance the meat has to travel, the better it is for you and for the environment. Organic practices require livestock to live outside at least part of the year and forage for a certain percentage of their diet. This more natural lifestyle leads to proteins that are higher in beneficial omega-3s, about 50 percent higher, and lower in omega-6s. I know it can be expensive to buy this type of meat, but if you want to save on costs, look for dark meat chicken (such as chicken legs and thighs), tougher cuts of beef for slow-cooking, and wild-caught fish on sale.

Fish: Choose wild-caught, lower-mercury seafood. Enjoy two six-ounce servings per week of the lowest mercury sources such as clams, crab (domestic), haddock, mackerel (North Atlantic, chub), oysters, salmon, sardines, scallops, and trout (freshwater). For a reference guide on the mercury content of fish, refer to https://www.ewg.org/consumer-guides/ewgs-consumer-guide -seafood.

Eggs: I recommend free-range and organic eggs.

Vegetables and Fruits: Purchase local and organic whenever possible. Nonorganic produce has varying degrees of pesticide residue. Eating foods that contain toxins stresses the liver by making it work harder to process and clear them from the body. If you cannot buy organic all the time, shop for conventional foods that are on the Clean Fifteen list of the Environmental Working Group (EWG), the top fifteen fruits and veggies that can be purchased conventional, if needed. Foods on the EWG's Dirty Dozen should be bought organic to avoid pesticides as much as possible. (Access the most up-to-date versions of these lists at ewg.org.)

Non-Dairy "Milk" Products: There is a wide variety of non-dairy (and soy-free) "milk" products now available at most grocery stores. Look for ones that are organic when possible, without additives such as carrageenan and gums.

Nuts and Seeds: Opt for raw, organic nuts and seeds. This way, you can sprout them if needed (sprouting increases the amount of antioxidants and reduces the amount of antinutrients such as phytic acid), and there are no added oils or salt that may do more harm than good. (When nuts and seeds are roasted, oftentimes

> inflammatory oils and iodine-treated salt are used, so it's best to
> buy them raw and make your own.)
>
> For a Shopping List and Kitchen Makeover Guide go to:
> thyroidpharmacist.com/atpbookbonus.

Add Gut-Supporting Foods

The following foods lower inflammation by nourishing your gut, promoting a healthy gut microbiome, and strengthening the gut wall. Try adding them regularly to your diet.

Fermented foods

Fermentation is a process of food preservation that produces probiotics, or "good" bacteria, that can balance intestinal flora and help with symptoms of constipation, digestion, and anxiety. Some of my favorite fermented foods include fermented coconut yogurt, fermented coconut water, and fermented cabbage. (Avoid malt vinegar, as it's made from barley, a gluten-containing grain.) Look in the refrigerated section of the grocery store, as these fermented foods will have the most probiotic bacteria.

Bone broth

Bone broth contains an abundance of healing minerals and amino acids, including collagen and gelatin, to support our gut lining, immune system, joint health, and skin. Gelatin in bone broth can help seal the junctions in the intestines so that they are no longer permeable. In doing so, pesky substances can no longer pass through the intestinal wall. This promotes gut healing and, in turn, reduces food sensitivities. It's also good for blood sugar balance and may counteract some of the negative effects of dietary fructose (sugar) consumption. Making your own can be easy and quick (see my slow cooker Bone Broth recipe on page 305)!

Fiber

Fiber acts like a sponge as it moves through the digestive system and helps absorb toxins and excess hormones, ultimately supporting their path to excretion. Recent research has also linked fiber to a healthy microbiome filled with "good" bacteria, critical for overall gut health and maintaining a strong intestinal lining. It's best to get fiber from fruits and vegetables rather than supplements (unless you are utilizing a specific gut-healing protocol) because fiber supplements have been known to aggravate intestinal permeability and SIBO (small intestinal bacterial overgrowth). I suggest gradually adding fibrous foods into your diet if you don't normally eat a lot of them.

SUPPLEMENT SPOTLIGHT #3: *SACCHAROMYCES BOULARDII*

Another important supplement I recommend for reducing inflammation is *Saccharomyces boulardii*. *S. boulardii* is one of my favorite supplements because of its extensive adrenal, gut, and immune system benefits. I first learned about the benefits of *S. boulardii* firsthand as a young pharmacist with a case of not-so-glamorous traveler's diarrhea. It is a gentle, beneficial yeast (also known as a probiotic yeast) that is often recommended to people who take antibiotics. (Probiotics like this one can help restore the balance of "good" bacteria after a course of antibiotics.)

S. boulardii boosts secretory IgA, or SIgA, the respiratory and gastrointestinal tracts' first line of defense. It can prevent the adhesion of parasites, bacteria, viruses, and other inflammatory pathogens to our respiratory and gut lining. This means that the body is better able to clear out and defend against chronic infections, including opportunistic and pathogenic organisms from the gut such as *Helicobacter pylori, Blastocystis hominis* (a common trigger for Hashimoto's), yeast overgrowth/*Candida*, and SIBO (small intestinal bacterial overgrowth), a common yet often hidden cause of leaky gut and inflammation.

But you don't need to have a gut infection to benefit from *S. boulardii*. Because it neutralizes toxins and decreases pathogens, *S. boulardii* reduces inflammation caused by an overactive immune response in the digestive system and helps set up a healthy microbiome. By helping to raise secretory IgA, *S. boulardii* has been shown to restore and strengthen the junctions between the cells that line the small intestine and even decrease leaky gut. One study that examined the impact of *S. boulardii* on cells taken from the colons of people with inflammatory bowel disease (IBD) found that the *S. boulardii* protected the epithelial cells (surface tissue) and improved the adhesion of one cell to another. This led to the overall restoration and strengthening of intestinal barrier function.

I have found that adding in *S. boulardii* can address the gut inflammation so common in adrenal dysfunction and autoimmune thyroiditis, while also improving skin issues, brain fog, anxiety, and joint pain.

I recommend 250 mg (5 billion CFU or colony-forming units, which indicates the number of live organisms in each dose), two times daily, at breakfast and dinner. Start low and go slow. If you experience symptoms such as bloating, nausea, dizziness, and diarrhea, cut back to one capsule per day, and if you are still experiencing digestive discomfort, trim back to half a capsule per day and then increase every three to five days. If intolerable symptoms persist, discontinue the supplement. You may require more gut healing before using this supplement comfortably.

It's important to note that many over-the-counter probiotics come in low concentrations, which are not enough to rebalance the gut. Other versions need to be kept in the fridge and are easily forgotten. This is why I included a heat-stable version of *S. boulardii* in my Rootcology supplement line. Rootcology *S. Boulardii* does not require refrigeration and has the ability to survive passage through the harsh gastric environment, withstanding high acidity, bile, and heat. Other high-potency options include Designs for Health Floramyces and Pure Encapsulations Saccharomyces boulardii.

Safety Signal #3: Balanced Blood Sugar

Wild swings in blood sugar put stress on the body and contribute to adrenal dysfunction, and this can often feel like fatigue, irritability, anger, or anxiety. Balancing my blood sugar was hugely transformative for me, and many of my clients report that balancing their blood sugar was the most helpful element of the program in taking back their health. You, too, can make a huge difference in your symptoms by adjusting your nutrition and incorporating habits that help maintain steady blood sugar balance throughout the day.

Use Food to Stabilize Blood Sugar

People with adrenal issues usually have hypoglycemia, and modifying our intake and frequency of macronutrients can remedy this. To understand how to keep our blood sugar stable, it helps to know how the body processes various types of macronutrients.

The glycemic index (GI) is a measure of how quickly food becomes assimilated into our bodies. It can also be referred to as the "burn" rate, or how quickly we burn the fuel we receive from these foods. Focusing on foods that "burn" slower can really help with balancing blood sugars.

The graphic on the following page gives you an idea of how low and high GI foods affect blood sugar over a two-hour period. As you can see, low GI foods produce a small spike that declines relatively slowly. In contrast, high GI foods send blood sugar levels soaring and then crashing (and burning) dramatically after thirty minutes.

Different macronutrient categories tend to have similar burn rates. Sugars and starches (carbohydrates) have a very fast burn rate, and thus can spike blood sugar levels dramatically. This quick assimilation can make us

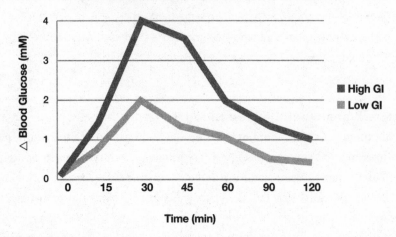

Blood Sugar Elevation Following Consumption of High GI or Low GI Foods

feel hungry again less than an hour after eating them. Fats and proteins have a slower burn rate and don't raise blood sugar levels as quickly, so you stay fuller longer.

Food and Hunger Guide

Type of Food	Time Until You Are Hungry Again
Carbohydrate	Forty-five minutes to one hour
Protein	Two to three hours
Fat	Four hours

Minimizing carbohydrates and eating frequent meals that are full of fat and protein will stabilize blood sugar levels, keep you feeling fuller longer, and can also improve your mood. In the early stages of blood sugar balance, I recommend eating every three hours.

Hanger Management

The blood sugar–balancing strategies will gradually work to bring your blood sugar swings under control and prevent high blood sugar and the "hanger"-inducing low blood sugar (hypoglycemia). In the long term, this will stabilize your mood and energy levels, but if you have low cortisol, you may find yourself with hypoglycemia that may take a while to stabilize when you start the program. Because cortisol and glucose have an intricate feedback system and often follow a similar circadian pattern, those with low cortisol tend to have low glucose around the same times of day. Feeling faint, confused, or light-headed after waking up and in the morning are potential signs that you are having low blood sugar.

For this reason, I have included orange juice in the morning Adrenal Kick Start recipe (page 297) so you can get a lift of blood glucose first thing in the morning. I have combined it with protein and coconut milk to get the benefits of the juice without a big crash, and the juice is followed by a smoothie about an hour later.

However, for acute low blood sugar situations, you may need a more quick-acting remedy for low blood sugar. In that case, drink 4 ounces of a fruit juice such as orange, apple, or grape juice. This will raise your glucose levels within ten to fifteen minutes. Please note that juices work faster than whole fruit because fiber in the fruit can slow down the absorption.

Practical Tips for Balancing Blood Sugar

- **Never skip breakfast:** Breakfast is the most important opportunity to set ourselves up for a successful day by replenishing nutrients and balancing our blood sugar.
- **Avoid most foods in boxes or packages:** These include cookies, cakes, crackers, candy, granola bars, sodas, pasta, breakfast cereals, and most ready-to-eat foods that have highly processed carbs.
- **Avoid fruit juice on its own:** Most fruit juices are loaded with quick-burning sugar. Instead, we'll opt for fruit/vegetable juices blended with healthy fats or pair juice with a meal that includes enough fat and/or protein (unless you are acutely hypoglycemic).
- **Consume low-glycemic "sweet" fruit in moderation (one or two servings per day):** Low-glycemic "sweet" fruits include blueberries, strawberries, raspberries, green apples, plums, pomegranate, cranberries, and oranges.
- **Include (healthy) fats and protein with every meal/snack:** When you do eat carbohydrates, combine them with fat or protein to minimize

the blood sugar surge. I recommend a ratio of no larger than two servings of carbohydrates to one serving of protein to ensure that the overall glycemic load of your meal stays low. For example, if you are having 4 ounces of steak, you should have a maximum of 8 ounces of sweet potatoes.

- **Utilize the benefits of low-glycemic "non-sweet" fruit:** These fruits include grapefruit (which can boost cortisol); avocados (an excellent source of good fat); and lemons, limes, and tomatoes (rich in adrenal-supporting vitamin C).

- **Consume starchy vegetables in moderation (one or two servings per day):** Be mindful not to overindulge in vegetables such as sweet potatoes and butternut squash. I suggest avoiding white potatoes because of how significantly they can raise blood sugar—almost as much as pure glucose!

- **Low-carb snacks:** Eating small, low-carb snacks rich in protein and fat every two to three hours will help with blood sugar balance and replenish nutrients. Think nuts, seeds, hard-boiled eggs, and protein shakes! (There are plenty of yummy snack suggestions included in the Recipes section. ☺)

- **Add cinnamon:** Studies have shown that cinnamon can slow the rate of carbohydrate breakdown in the digestive tract and moderate rises in blood sugar levels. I also recommend pumpkin pie spice (a blend of ground cinnamon, nutmeg, ginger, cloves, and allspice) as a tasty ingredient to stabilize blood sugar. You can add it to your smoothies, gluten-free baked goods, and even hot beverages!

- **Eat on a schedule:** Many of us forget to eat until we are "hangry." In the beginning of the program, in order to rebalance the body's hunger pathways, we will eat every two to three hours. (See A Sample Day on the Adrenal Transformation Protocol on page 245.)

  - We will start the day with the easy-to-digest energizing Adrenal Kick Start (page 297) within thirty minutes of waking, followed by a breakfast smoothie one hour later.

  - We will incorporate snacks/caffeine-free lattes/teas/green juices in between breakfast and lunch to help with balancing blood sugar, hunger hormones, and energy levels and resetting the circadian rhythm (see more below) through increased daytime caloric intake.

- We will schedule a nourishing and balancing midday lunch, followed by another choice of snacks/lattes/teas/green juices two to three hours later to prevent the afternoon slump. As Julie A. said: "That 3 p.m. latte snack was a game changer. No more 3 p.m. slump!"
- An easy-to-digest dinner is scheduled for the early evening to set us up for a restful sleep.
- At the beginning of the program, we will have an option for an after-dinner snack/tea to support restful sleep through stable blood sugar levels at night.

This schedule works wonders for fatigue, and by the end of the program, participants feel more energetic and satisfied and are able to move toward a healthier weight. Over time, participants following a nourishing, blood sugar–balancing diet with supplements are able to extend the periods between food.

SUPPLEMENT SPOTLIGHT #4: MYO-INOSITOL

Myo-inositol is an important nutrient and type of natural sugar alcohol found in many plants and animals. It regulates several critical functions and hormones associated with adrenal, endocrine, and thyroid health and has been shown to have anti-inflammatory and antioxidant properties.

Studies suggest that myo-inositol can help maintain good blood sugar balance by increasing insulin sensitivity. It can also help with the mood swings, anxiety, and obsessive-compulsive disorder (OCD) associated with stressed-out adrenals and fluctuating thyroid hormones. This may be due to its involvement in stimulating the production of the "feel-good" hormone serotonin. Personally I recommend myo-inositol to clients, as I believe that, at least for some people, it offers effective support for anxiety, OCD, sleep problems, and more.

Myo-inositol also brings menstrual health and fertility benefits. In studies of women with PCOS, supplementing with myo-inositol was shown to improve ovarian function, the pregnancy rate, and the quality of embryos.

Additionally, it provides thyroid health support with supplementation shown to reduce thyroid antibodies, reduce TSH levels, and even achieve remission in people with Hashimoto's. A 2017 study confirmed these earlier findings, noting that thyroid antibodies, TSH, and quality of life were all significantly improved after administration of both myo-inositol and selenium (a nutrient proven to be effective at reducing thyroid antibodies). Interestingly, there was one case of hyperthyroidism included in this study, and in that single case, the supplementation increased TSH levels up to normal concentrations.

Our bodies can produce myo-inositol, but research suggests that some people may not be able to meet their body's metabolic needs through synthesis alone. While adding more foods such as blueberries (which are rich in the nutrient) to your diet is one way of getting more myo-inositol (check out the recipe for Blueberry Pie Smoothie, page 303), keep in mind that if you have poor digestive abilities, like most people with adrenal dysfunction, poor nutrient absorption can make it challenging to get enough.

Supplementing with myo-inositol will help you get enough of this important nutrient and also help you with other root causes and symptoms. Because I've seen so many mood- and hormone-balancing benefits with myo-inositol, I developed Rootcology Myo-Inositol Powder, a naturally sweet-tasting powder that dissolves easily. I love stirring it into a cup of tea for a hint of sweetness. I recommend ¼ teaspoon (700 mg), once per day, after dinner. Other high-quality myo-inositol supplements I like are Designs for Health Inositol Powder and Pure Encapsulations Inositol (powder).

Thyroid Tip: Combining myo-inositol with selenium can improve thyroid function and reduce thyroid antibodies. You can add Pure Encapsulations Selenium 200 mcg to the myo-inositol in the program or replace the myo-inositol powder with Rootcology's Myo-Inositol + Selenium blend, which contains 600 mg of myo-inositol and 83 mcg of selenium, the thyroid-beneficial dose used in most studies. Be sure to follow up with your doctor to test your lab values after initiating myo-inositol, as it can lower or eliminate your need for thyroid medications.

PCOS SOS: Combining myo-inositol with D-chiro-inositol can improve ovarian function and normalize menses. You can add D-chiro-inositol to the myo-inositol in the program as a stand-alone supplement (100 mg to 1,000 mg per day, Klaire Labs and Neurobiologix brands), or you can replace Rootcology Myo-Inositol with Ovasitol (2,000 mg myo-inositol/50 mg D-chiro-inositol twice per day), the dose combination that has been studied to be the most helpful. Sensitol by Designs for Health is also an option.

ATP SUCCESS STORIES

"This program helped me balance my blood sugar levels. I did not realize how much sugar I was consuming and [am] so happy to no longer crave sugar. . . . I feel I've made a lot of progress eliminating sugar, grains, and dairy."—KRISTEN K.

"I started eliminating all bread, grains, and dairy on day 1 of the program . . . The following day I awoke for the first time without mucus congestion in my sinuses and chest. My acid reflux diminished within 2 days and is now gone altogether."—JENNIFER W.

"I cut out sugar (sweets and treats). . . . I recommitted to going gluten- and dairy-free when I started the program and I feel so much better. No cravings so far, which is a miracle in itself, plus I've been so much nicer to my kids. I don't feel like I'm trapped on an emotional roller coaster every day. I've already lost about 5 pounds and my clothes are fitting better. My skin looks healthier too. I can't wait to see how I feel at the end of the program!"—LAUREN V.

"I have more energy once I drink the kick start/smoothie in the mornings. . . . This program really helped me realize different ways that the timing of when you eat and what you eat can make such a difference in symptoms such as fatigue and energy. Also, there is so much more to our health than diet, supplements, and exercise. I struggle with mindset and this aspect of my health, but this program really helps break it down into tangible steps for how to help your body remember how to heal itself. Blood sugar balance is something I didn't realize was so pivotal in feeling energy and less fatigue. I think that was really eye opening for me."—MAGDA B.

Action Steps

To get the most nourishment and replenishment, aim to:

- Stock your kitchen with an abundance of nutrient-rich foods—and clear out the high-glycemic, inflammatory foods inhibiting your healing.
- Keep it simple: Use the recipes in this book to start making tasty, no-fuss smoothies, meals, and snacks.
- Add core supplements to your routine. If you choose to add only one, make it an adrenal-balancing supplement with the ABCs: a mixture of adaptogenic herbs, B vitamins, and vitamin C.

To view the scientific references cited in this chapter, please visit us online at https://thyroidpharmacist.com/atpbooknotes.

Reenergize

Goals

- Accomplish daily tasks with energy and ease through proper electrolyte balance and hydration.
- Feel more focused, energized, and clear-headed during the day.
- Get more high-quality, restorative sleep at night.

Fatigue is one of the most common and debilitating symptoms people with adrenal dysfunction report. It can make you feel like you are dragging around fifty pounds of concrete, especially in the later phases of adrenal fatigue when your cortisol becomes depleted. I know firsthand how tiredness and fatigue can impact everyday life and leave you exhausted. Before I healed my adrenals, I needed to sleep for twelve hours each night to be able to function . . . and by "function," I mean, after hitting the snooze button on my alarm clock for two hours (ask my poor husband), I would drag myself out of bed and then had to drink four to six cups of caffeine every day to keep myself awake. I often had Red Bull and Pepsi for breakfast and was the epitome of "wired but tired." Overcoming fatigue is an important step in healing your adrenals and getting on with life, and the safety signals in this chapter are intended to help with that by restoring your energy.

Food pharmacology can do a lot to reenergize us. Using food and targeted supplementation to meet the body's nutritional needs, lower inflammation, and balance blood sugar in alignment with the three safety signals we covered in the previous chapter will help energy levels to bounce back, but there's still more we can do. You'll discover that to overcome fatigue and other adrenal-related symptoms, *when* we eat and perform certain daily activities is just as important as *what* we eat.

To help us feel more vibrant and alive during the day and relaxed and able to get good sleep at night, we'll add circadian timing to the power of nutrition to send the following safety signals to our body:

1. **Hydration:** Proper hydration is so important to all of the body's cells and systems that we can only survive a few days without water (but can go weeks without food!). Dehydration impairs the production of ATP, our main energy molecule, decreases blood flow to the muscles and brain, and disrupts the sleep cycle, leaving us feeling drained, weak, brain foggy, and irritable. Paying attention to adequate salt and hydration status during the day, especially in the morning (but not too much at night), can help bring back energy and homeostasis in the body by supporting healthy blood pressure and cortisol levels—and prevent the need to run to the potty in the middle of the night!

2. **Mitochondrial support:** Just like there are numerous reasons for inflammation, there are numerous reasons why we may have mitochondrial dysfunction. I think of the mitochondria as enigmatic little creatures that are delicate, yet oh so powerful. They need the optimal circumstances to do their powerful work of producing adrenal hormones and ATP. Because the body is a system, supporting mitochondria can send safety signals clearing the way for healthy energy levels and reduced brain fog.

3. **Circadian rhythm reset:** Timing matters when it comes to providing the body what it needs to heal. When we get the wrong kind of light or eat the wrong foods at the wrong times, our body can sense this as stress. We will prioritize timing daily habits, including when we eat and the consumption of strategic foods and supplements, to align with our circadian rhythm and promote healthy levels of cortisol and energy throughout the day.

The healing and energizing benefits of two supplements offer added support:

- An electrolyte blend to maintain good fluid balance, reduce inflammation, and reset the circadian rhythm.
- Carnitine to promote energy, blood sugar balance, and the function of the mitochondria.

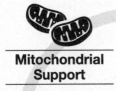
Mitochondrial Support

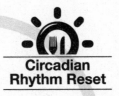
Circadian Rhythm Reset

Reenergize

Rebalance Hydration

Safety Signal #1: Hydration

Hydration may not be the first thing you think of when it comes to adrenal health, but proper hydration with water and electrolytes is a key component to healing, and 93 percent of members who tried the hydration strategies in the program found them to be helpful! So, how much water should you drink?

The general recommendation is 6 to 8 cups (or 6 to 8 eight-ounce glasses) per day of clean, filtered water. But to get a precise amount specific for your body, use this simple calculation:

Your body weight in pounds ÷ 2 = your daily water intake in ounces

For example, if you weigh 150 pounds, you would aim to drink 75 ounces of water per day, although of course your individual needs may vary. To make sure you're drinking sufficient water, you may find it helpful to keep track of your water intake in your health journal or with a free water counting app on your smartphone.

If you've gotten bored of plain water, kick the flavor up a notch by adding fruit, vegetables, and herbs. I like to add one of these blends to a pitcher of water and sip throughout the day:

- Strawberry, cucumber, and mint
- Lemon and lime
- Basil and orange

Or, find your own favorite flavor combination!

It's important to note that water is just one piece of the hydration puzzle. We may also need electrolytes.

One community member named Kate thought she was drinking enough water to keep her hydrated but noticed a significant improvement in her symptoms and energy once she started intentionally replenishing her electrolytes. She shared, "My chiropractor was always telling me 'You're dehydrated' and I was like, how? I drink a ton of water. Well apparently I was [dehydrated]! The Electrolyte Blend gave me calm. No more heart palpitations and I am 'regular' for the first time in my life! Adding the electrolyte blend is the only change I have made. I have more energy . . . [and] I would think this is a huge help to my busted adrenals as well since I feel calm. Thank you!"

Electrolytes

You may think only athletes need to replenish electrolytes to stay hydrated, but those of us with adrenal dysfunction and hypothyroidism are often deficient in these nutrients and stand to gain physical and mental stamina by maintaining adequate levels. With an impaired stress response, just getting through your day can feel like running a marathon! Restoring electrolyte balance can help make everyday tasks much easier.

A word of caution, however, is that a lot of electrolyte products, including sports drinks such as Gatorade, are not necessarily healthy options because of their high levels of sugar, dyes, and flavorings. A little bit of natural sugar in an electrolyte supplement is okay, since glucose helps the body absorb the electrolyte minerals. I recommend choosing a supplement blend that replenishes the body's main electrolytes, such as sodium, chloride, magnesium, and potassium.

Electrolytes, such as sodium and potassium, are minerals in your body that help the body function. They support muscle health by ensuring that our muscles contract properly (hint: muscle cramping and soreness may be a sign of poor electrolyte balance!), maintain fluid balance within the body, and play critical roles in digestive, nervous system, and cardiovascular health, especially regarding blood pressure regulation.

This is why low blood pressure often accompanies adrenal imbalance. When we have an electrolyte imbalance, we can become dehydrated, and we may experience symptoms such as fatigue, a fast heartbeat, diarrhea, or constipation. Electrolytes can help us feel focused and energized, mentally and physically, so it's important that we take steps to replenish them.

Electrolytes can be found in a variety of foods, including meat and fish, bone broths, fruits and vegetables, sea salt, sea vegetables, and teas. It's important to know that sodium seems to be the most important electrolyte in terms of adrenal balance, so I recommend focusing on sodium-rich electrolytes, in the form of high-quality sea salt. The kind of salt is very important. Avoid salt that is processed and/or fortified with iodine ("iodized" salt) and opt for high-quality sea salt instead. The following types of sea salt may contain very low levels of iodine but are mainly composed of sodium and trace minerals:

- Pink Himalayan sea salt
- Gray Himalayan sea salt
- Celtic/Mediterranean white sea salt

THYROID TIP

Although iodine deficiency can lead to iodine-deficiency hypothyroidism, this type of hypothyroidism is not common. High iodine intake has been shown to exacerbate Hashimoto's, the most common cause of hypothyroidism.

SODIUM AND POTASSIUM MODIFICATIONS FOR CORTISOL AND BLOOD PRESSURE

While sodium-rich salt has health benefits, individuals with hypertension, Ménière's disease, diabetes, vascular dementia, and asthma should check with their doctors before consuming high levels of salt. Remember, while in the advanced stages of adrenal dysfunction, people tend to have low blood pressure and low cortisol (and salt can increase both).

In the early stages of adrenal dysfunction, people are more likely to have water retention, high cortisol, and high blood pressure. Be sure to listen to your body. In some cases, listening may involve using a blood pressure cuff. ☺

Low Cortisol	Cortisol Roller Coaster	High Cortisol
Add more salt to your diet to stretch out cortisol and support blood pressure in the morning and early afternoon.	Consider adding more salt if you have morning/afternoon fatigue, but avoid salt if you have high blood pressure.	Avoid adding more salt to your diet, as it can increase your cortisol levels and blood pressure further.

Sodium and potassium, another important electrolyte, work together to maintain balance in the body. If sodium levels are dysregulated, potassium levels are likely to be so as well. You may need *MORE* potassium if you experience:

- Excessive thirst
- Salt cravings
- Water retention
- Cognitive issues
- High blood pressure
- Heartbeat fluctuations
- Nervousness

You may need *LESS* potassium if you:

- Have low blood pressure
- Are on a potassium chloride supplement
- Experience GI symptoms such as nausea or vomiting

If you are experiencing any of these symptoms, I recommend getting a blood test done for your potassium levels to see if either of these hydration blends is optimal for you.

Hydration Blends
Less Potassium
1 quart filtered water
½ teaspoon sea salt (white, gray, or pink)

More Potassium
1 quart coconut water
¼ to ½ teaspoon sea salt (white, gray, or pink)

How to incorporate electrolytes into your daily routine:
- Sprinkle sea salt on food at each meal, to taste.
- Add salt to your drinking water or other diet-friendly beverages throughout the day. I recommend starting your day with my Adrenal Kick Start (page 297), which includes a healthy sprinkle!
- Make Sole (recipe on page 301), a high-concentration mixture of Himalayan sea salt and filtered water. This salt mixture can be taken once per day, up to 1 teaspoon at a time, diluted in water, on an empty stomach or in recipes.
- Go with your cravings unless you have a medical reason not to do so. People with adrenal issues will often crave salt, what I like to call the "I just ate a whole bag of chips" syndrome. So you can have that salt you crave if you choose that high-quality sea salt!
- Drink plenty of bone broth, a high-electrolyte food. Try my recipe on page 305.

- Utilize my sodium and potassium hydration blends in the Sodium and Potassium Modifications for Cortisol and Blood Pressure box on page 154.
- Last but not least, utilize the Electrolyte Blend. (See Supplement Spotlight #5.)

SUPPLEMENT SPOTLIGHT #5: ELECTROLYTE BLEND

I developed Rootcology Electrolyte Blend as a complete and balanced electrolyte formula, boosted with adrenal support powerhouse ingredients to support hydration status in people with adrenal dysfunction (and everyone else, too). This formula contains the electrolytes sodium, potassium, chloride, and magnesium, along with:

- **Vitamin C:** A high dose of vitamin C that helps with adrenal function, immunity, the mitochondria, thyroid hormones, and collagen production.
- **Quercetin/rutin/citrus bioflavonoids:** These work synergistically with vitamin C and reduce inflammation. They also have antihistamine and antiviral properties.
- **Taurine:** An amino acid that supports the gallbladder, helps remove fluoride from the body, aids digestion, helps with allergies, and supports healthy blood pressure through electrolyte regulation in the cells.
- **D-ribose:** A natural sugar, D-ribose supports our hydration status and exercise recovery. I chose it because studies in athletes doing high-intensity training revealed significant improvements in performance, reduced muscle damage, and a lowered perceived exertion. While I don't recommend intense training with adrenal dysfunction, I do recommend D-ribose, as it can help with fatigue and exertion caused by day-to-day life tasks. (After all, running errands can feel like a major athletic endeavor for many with adrenal dysfunction!)

You can drink the electrolytes in water, or you can upgrade your Adrenal Kick Start drink (page 297) by switching up the salt for a scoop of electrolytes in the recipe. I like to add a scoop to my smoothie for a refreshing citrus flavor.

Designs for Health's Electrolyte Synergy is another comprehensive blend that I like, as well as Pure Encapsulations Electrolyte/Energy Formula. If utilizing the Electrolyte/Energy Formula, I recommend adding a stand-alone D-ribose supplement, such as Pure Encapsulations.

Please note that electrolyte imbalances may be compounded by intense exercise, living in a hot or dry climate, and drinking caffeine or alcohol. If any of these are true for you, you may need more water and electrolytes than you think.

Fibromyalgia and CFS Success: Doses of 250 mg to 15 grams of D-ribose per day have been studied for various conditions, such as fibromyalgia and chronic fatigue syndrome (CFS). The Rootcology Electrolytes contain around 700 mg, and for best results you may wish to add more D-ribose if you have one of these conditions.

What About Caffeine?

We should probably talk about the elephant in the room . . . caffeine intake and the adrenals! Too much caffeine can weaken our adrenals by triggering the stress response and increasing the production of adrenal hormones, including cortisol. Caffeine lowers our insulin sensitivity so that our cells no longer respond to insulin properly and blood sugar levels remain high. High blood sugar is perceived as a stress by the body, raising cortisol levels.

In the early stages of adrenal dysfunction, caffeine can exacerbate high cortisol, and as the adrenal dysfunction progresses to a low-cortisol state as time goes on, we may become dependent on caffeine to get a boost of cortisol. The caffeine helps keep us going, but as our adrenals become weaker, we tend to get more stressed out and anxious. Our quality of sleep suffers and without enough rest, we're likely to reach for a caffeinated beverage—or two or three. And the cycle starts all over again: caffeine, weaker adrenals, more caffeine, even weaker adrenals.

Caffeine also increases gut permeability, further contributing to adrenal dysfunction.

So why isn't caffeine part of the "excluded" foods for the program? I've come to realize that while reliance on caffeine for enough energy to make it through the day may exacerbate adrenal dysfunction, it's not usually the cause of adrenal dysfunction; rather, it's a consequence.

Asking fatigued people to quit caffeine without providing tools to support their daytime energy levels can lead to an exacerbation of adrenal symptoms like mood instability and fatigue and can cause even the most committed people to "fall off the wagon" and sabotage their entire healing protocol because they were unable to function without caffeine.

Additionally, caffeine is an addictive substance, so some people may get withdrawal headaches, fatigue, nausea, irritability, diarrhea, and even vomiting if they quit cold turkey instead of weaning off gradually—especially if they have a history of consuming a lot of caffeine for a long time (this is not a theory; this is something I learned the hard way).

Instead of asking you to quit cold turkey, the ATP strategies will help you increase your energy naturally, which will help reduce your dependence on caffeine over time. If you currently drink more than two cups of tea or coffee a day, and especially if you drink caffeine after noon, I do encourage you to make a gradual reduction plan, and consider moving your caffeine intake to earlier times in the day. ATP participants have shared:

"For the first time in years, I was actually able to wean from caffeine without the nasty withdrawal side effects!"

"I was able to completely wean off of caffeine and cut out all sugar sources without any issue."

HOW TO GRADUALLY REDUCE CAFFEINE INTAKE

To wean off caffeine, I recommend a gradual reduction method over the course of four weeks, where caffeine is reduced by 25 percent of the initial intake each week. I generally recommend starting this process after being on the program for at least one week and having incorporated some of the energy-building methods outlined in this chapter.

Here's a sample plan for a person who started off drinking 4 cups of coffee per day.

- Before Week 1: 4 cups per day
- After Week 1: 3 cups per day
- After Week 2: 2 cups per day
- After Week 3: 1 cup per day
- After Week 4: wean off

If you are thinking about quitting caffeine, the following strategies will help reduce your withdrawal:

- Give the circadian ATP diet and supplement strategies a week or so to work before reducing caffeine intake.
- Use Epsom salt baths to help prevent and reduce headaches.
- Consider "coffee replacement beverages" that combine adaptogens with lower amounts of caffeine. Please be sure to cross-reference the adaptogens in your supplements and food products to make sure you don't take excessive doses of adaptogens.
  - MUD\WTR, made with black tea and adaptogenic mushrooms (most compatible with Rootcology and Pure Encapsulations Adrenal Support Blends)
  - Four Sigmatic Mushroom Coffee, various blends of coffee and different adaptogens
  - Rasa Coffee Alternative (contains some overlapping ingredients to Rootcology and Pure Encapsulations Adrenal Support Blends, so only use as a replacement)
- Consider gentle detox-promoting beverages:
  - Dandy Blend: This instant herbal beverage is a great-tasting substitute for coffee. Made with dandelion, it is a gluten- and

caffeine-free alternative to coffee that gently supports the body's detox pathways to minimize coffee withdrawal symptoms. Dandy indeed!

- Lemon water: In the morning, freshly squeeze the juice of ½ to 1 organic lemon in 1 cup of hot water, and drink it for an energy boost.
- Consider caffeine-free Balancing Teas (page 161).

Experience the Healing Properties of Tea

At the beginning of each week, my team and I meet to discuss the week ahead. If you asked any of my team members what they remember most about me from that meeting, I suspect they would say my fancy mug filled to the brim with herbal tea! I love tea and hope you'll come to love it, too. During the program, I encourage you to try drinking a mug or two a day.

Tea has long been associated with good health and medicinal properties and now numerous studies have shown that different varieties of tea contain stress-relieving, anti-inflammatory, and immune-strengthening properties, among others. There are so many different kinds of tea available, each boasting its own distinctive delicious flavor and unique healing benefits.

For the ATP, we'll focus on caffeine-free herbal teas (made from a plant's flowers, fruit, leaves, seeds, or roots) that support the adrenals and thyroid. For my favorite relaxing tea options, see Balancing Teas on page 161. They can be prepared as directed on the package and sipped on as desired, throughout the day. Each afternoon, I like to amplify the healing powers of tea by drinking it as part of a daily stress-relieving ritual. I take a few moments to slowly sip a mug in a quiet place, reflect on my intentions, and feel the stress of the day ease away. Rituals help us to relax because our brains and bodies know what to expect.

Do note the precautions for each tea, and always be sure to speak with your healthcare provider if you are taking any medications, are pregnant or breastfeeding, or have preexisting health conditions (see Balancing Teas [page 161] for information on specific teas).

BALANCING TEAS

Tea	Description	Precautions
Chamomile for better sleep and relaxation	Compounds such as flavonoids and apigenin lend chamomile its sleep-inducing properties by activating "sleep mode" within the brain.	—Should not be used by those who are sensitive to the Asteraceae/ Compositae family. —Avoid if you have conditions that may worsen with estrogen exposure. —Avoid in pregnancy. —May increase milk supply in breastfeeding moms.
Lemon balm for anxiety support	Active compounds in lemon balm may promote the production of GABA (gamma-aminobutyric acid), a neurotransmitter that helps regulate mood imbalances and reduces stress and anxiety.	—Should not be used by women who are pregnant. —May reduce milk supply while breastfeeding.
Tulsi/holy basil throughout the day to support healthy cortisol levels and for reducing anxiety	An adaptogen that helps the body become more resilient to stress. Its mood-stabilizing effects have been compared to the antianxiety medication diazepam.	—Should not be used by those who are pregnant or trying to conceive due to contraceptive effects. —Used in herbal medicine by nursing moms as a galactagogue.
Passionflower in the evening for sleep, or to relieve anxiety	Promotes sleep and may lessen anxiety. One study found it can increase one's sleep time and sleep quality by promoting optimal amounts of REM and slow-wave sleep (both important for high-quality sleep).	—Should not be used by those who are pregnant or breastfeeding.

Tea	Description	Precautions
Licorice root for a morning energy boost	Helps increase cortisol production, resulting in a healthier stress response.	—Should not be used by those who have a history of high blood pressure, liver or kidney disease, or by those who are pregnant. —Women who are breastfeeding should consult with their doctor or midwife before using.
Rosehip for pain reduction	Rich in several compounds that contain powerful antioxidant properties, such as polyphenols and vitamins C and E, rosehip tea supports a healthy immune system, while galactolipids, the primary fat in cell membranes, have a strong anti-inflammatory effect shown to reduce pain.	—Should not be used by those who are pregnant or breastfeeding or have a history of deep-vein thrombosis, pulmonary embolisms, or other conditions involving clots.
Peppermint for digestive support	Exerts relaxing effects on the gastrointestinal system, promoting a "rest and digest" state that is crucial for optimal digestion.	—Speak with your practitioner if you have any preexisting conditions or are taking medications. —Avoid in pregnancy. —May suppress milk supply in women who are breastfeeding.
Ginger for digestive support	Ginger's antioxidant and anti-inflammatory properties reduce the oxidative damage that creates stress on the body and immune system.	—Should not be used by those with gallbladder disease or who are taking blood-thinning medications. —Avoid in pregnancy. —There are no known precautions for those who are breastfeeding, but it is always a good idea to check with your doctor.

Tea	Description	Precautions
Hibiscus for lowering blood pressure, blood sugar, and cholesterol	Rich in vitamin C, it also contains compounds such as phenols and flavonoids that act to reduce oxidative damage and strengthen the immune system.	—Avoid with low blood pressure and hypoglycemia. —Speak with your practitioner if you have any preexisting conditions or are taking medications. —There are no known precautions for those who are pregnant or breastfeeding, but it is always a good idea to check with your doctor.
Catnip for sleep and anxiety	Contains a compound called nepetalactone, which acts as a sedative, lending this herb its calming, stress-reducing qualities.	—Should not be used by those who are pregnant or breastfeeding or have pelvic inflammatory disease or heavy menstruation.

Safety Signal #2: Support the Mitochondria

A big transformation happened for me when I realized that caffeine was a way for people to self-medicate as a consequence of adrenal dysfunction rather than the cause of adrenal dysfunction. I was intrigued to learn that one of the underlying reasons why we may be dependent on caffeine is due to its ability to stimulate the mitochondria. The deeper I dove into the mitochondria, the more I realized that they are an important root cause for many issues, including adrenal dysfunction. Thus, in order to allow the body to get back to thriving and lose its dependence on caffeine, we need to properly support the mitochondria.

How the Adrenal Transformation Protocol Supports Mitochondria

If you are a nerd like me, you may have noticed that the abbreviation for this protocol is ATP (excuse me while I giggle, snort, and fix my glasses), and yes, this was intentional! You may remember the mitochondria as the site within the adrenals for making adrenal hormones, and the mitochondria also burn fatty acids from our diet and turn them into ATP. ATP (also known as adenosine triphosphate) is like the body's energy bank that is used for storing and transferring energy in cells, providing the fuel needed to run all of the body's systems.

Over time, chronic stress can damage the physical structure of the mitochondria as well as impair the way they work. When mitochondria become damaged or impaired and are no longer working optimally, we may experience low energy and fatigue and dysregulation of all of our adrenal hormones, including cortisol and estrogen—and the mood changes, low libido, and muscle weakness that can go along with it!

We'll be supporting the mitochondria on the ATP by making sure they have all of the nutrients they need to make energy efficiently and repair any physical damage.

Several of the diet and supplement strategies I've recommended as part of the Adrenal Transformation already have multitasking powers and are also necessary for the production of energy and healthy mitochondrial function:

- **Eating lots of fat:** The mitochondria require fatty acids from fats to make ATP, so a fat deficiency can actually cause energy deficiency.
- **B vitamins:** B vitamins keep the mitochondria running, acting as cofactors or coenzymes for all of the processes that occur in the mitochondria. If B vitamins run low, everything slows down.
- **Vitamin C:** Vitamin C is needed to break down fatty acids and turn them into energy.
- **Magnesium:** Magnesium helps mitochondria repair damage caused by stress, optimizing the production of energy.
- **Multitasking adaptogens:** Ashwagandha, eleuthero, and rhodiola rosea (included in the Rootcology Adrenal Support supplement) have been found to enhance mitochondrial function and work best in synergy as part of an adrenal support blend.
- **D-ribose:** In addition to being wonderful for hydration, D-ribose in the Rootcology Electrolyte Blend also helps support ATP production. (If you are using an electrolyte blend that does not contain D-ribose, you can get a stand-alone D-ribose supplement.)

Yet there's still more we can do! Carnitine is a key mitochondrial nutrient with multiple benefits; adding it to the mix can support the mitochondria and help turn the corner on exhaustion and cloudy thinking. See Supplement Spotlight #6.

SUPPLEMENT SPOTLIGHT #6: CARNITINE

So many of my clients come to me with fatigue, and carnitine supplementation is often a game-changer for them. It can really help boost energy, improve brain function, and support muscle strength. As one community member shared, "The debilitating fatigue I had before seems to be much better due to the carnitine supplement." I have personally seen people awaken from a brain-foggy "sloth mode" from carnitine supplementation, and my own postpartum muscle weakness, aches, and pains were reversed with carnitine! Research backs up my observations and experience, finding supplementation with L-carnitine improved fatigue. In one study, the most significant improvements were seen in "brain fatigue."

Carnitine optimizes the body's ability to burn fat for energy by transporting fatty acids into the mitochondria where they can be burned and used. This can help so much with blood sugar balance! Carnitine also removes toxic brain fog–inducing by-products like ammonia from the gut and promotes gut motility. All of this means more energy and less fatigue, less brain fog, less constipation, fewer digestive issues, and less muscle weakness and aches.

Although we can make most of the body's carnitine requirements under the right conditions, we also need to get it from diet, primarily meat and other animal products. The average adult diet offers about 75 percent of daily carnitine requirements (about 25 percent of the body's carnitine requirement is made by the body itself). Vegans and vegetarians generally don't consume enough carnitine, and research has found that their gut microbiota can become unable to adequately metabolize it. Even with a balanced, carnitine-rich diet, people with imbalanced adrenals or Hashimoto's may find it difficult to retain and/ or synthesize healthy levels of carnitine. Common issues associated with these conditions, such as nutrient deficiencies, inflammation, and digestive issues, impair the absorption of the B vitamins and vitamin C needed to make carnitine. In fact, carnitine deficiencies have been associated with thyroid imbalances and have been found in people with both hyperthyroid and hypothyroid conditions.

To make sure you're getting enough carnitine, start by ensuring that you are including good, clean sources of carnitine in your diet, like quality, hormone/antibiotic-free, organic meats. Red/dark meat (beef) is the highest source (3 ounces of beef steak contains 81 mg), followed by pork (3 ounces contain 24 mg); and significantly lower amounts can be found in fish and chicken.

You may be surprised to hear that more red meat may be beneficial in some cases, but in the case of energy production, it's true. It's amazing that when we remove inflammatory foods, we can really tune in to our bodies. My husband and I joked that I had a burger deficiency when I was pregnant, and the burgers were indeed an excellent source of not just iron but also carnitine, two commonly depleted nutrients in pregnancy.

In addition, I recommend a supplement to help maintain optimal carnitine levels and ensure you are supporting your mitochondria and metabolism. Carnitine comes in several forms, each with its own unique benefits.

- L-carnitine: May resolve fatigue and works to support antioxidant activities in the body. It is also essential for muscle functioning. In research, it has been shown to resolve muscle weakness and soreness and is often used in supplements intended for athletic performance improvements, optimal fat burning, and muscle recovery.
- Acetyl-L-carnitine: Considered more beneficial to the brain than L-carnitine and may help reduce mental fatigue (bye-bye, brain fog!).

Rootcology Carnitine Blend combines 400 mg of L-carnitine with 100 mg of acetyl-l-carnitine so that you get the benefits of both forms in one supplement. I recommend a dose of 1,000 mg of carnitine (ideally, a combination of these forms), twice per day. I also like Designs for Health Carnitine Synergy and Pure Encapsulations L-Carnitine, though the Pure Encapsulations L-Carnitine does not provide the acetylated form.

Beyond diet and supplements, the mitochondria also benefit from lifestyle changes that support circadian balance. When people hear about the circadian rhythm, they may think about sleep, but daytime exposure to natural outdoor light and darkness at night supports our energy levels in other ways. It allows us to make more of the hormone melatonin, which helps preserve mitochondrial function, and light helps the mitochondria make more energy. That's why the last and super-important way to let your body know it's safe and boost energy is by rebalancing the circadian rhythm.

Safety Signal #3: Circadian Rhythm Reset

Restoring circadian rhythm balance is about much more than improving sleep quality. In Chapter 2, I mentioned that sleep deprivation is the fastest way to induce HPA axis dysfunction, and as you may have guessed, getting plenty of sleep is one of the most helpful tools to rebalance the HPA axis. But while sleep is certainly a big part of the puzzle, the circadian rhythm is about much more than getting good rest. It is intimately tied to our adrenal function, mood, energy, and health. That's because the circadian rhythm, the body's biological clock, regulates several bodily functions, including daily fluctuations in sleeping and wakefulness, hormone release, body temperature, digestion, and metabolism.

When the circadian rhythm is functioning properly, it runs in sync with the twenty-four-hour day and the natural cycle of light and dark. Sunlight on our retinas sends signals to the brain that it's time to be up and awake and initiates several actions to "power up" the body for the day ahead, including activating morning cortisol production to help us hop out of bed alert and energized (peaking about one hour after waking), and signaling the digestive system to get ready for incoming nutrients.

The onset of darkness tells the brain that it's time for the body to start powering down to prepare for sleep, a time of rest and healing. Cortisol levels, slowly and steadily declining throughout the day, fall super low around bedtime, allowing us to feel tired so that we can fall asleep, and reach their lowest point around midnight. The digestive system slows down—why eating late at night can cause tummy troubles—and hormones that help the body grow and repair are released.

When this natural rhythm becomes disrupted, our energy levels and sleep are profoundly affected. We may experience daytime fatigue and all-around low energy, or a tired-but-wired feeling that makes it difficult to fall asleep at night, even when the body is exhausted. We may have trouble falling asleep or staying asleep; waking too early can happen as well. And then there are the digestive and immune issues, brain fog, mood swings, and low libido!

There are many reasons why the circadian rhythm can become unbalanced and a lot of them are linked to the artificial lights of modern living that make nighttime as bright as daytime, so the body doesn't get the "power down" message. These include the blue lights constantly emitted from electronic devices (cellphones, laptops, tablets). Studies have found that blue light can significantly impact the circadian rhythm, increase alertness, and contribute to sleep problems when used at night. Additionally, many of us spend much of our day indoors, away from natural sunlight in the morning and throughout the day. Other causes of circadian rhythm imbalance include:

- Overnight or off-hours work shifts
- Frequent changes in work shifts
- Travel over one or more time zones, a.k.a. jet lag
- Certain medications
- Sleep apnea, a condition that causes temporary periods where breathing stops during sleep. (Snoring is associated with sleep apnea, so if you snore, you may want to get tested. For more on sleep apnea, see Insomnia and Sleep Issues [page 273] in Chapter 10.)

Circadian rhythm imbalance is so common, but many of us don't even know that this is the reason behind our fatigue, irritability, insomnia, and fuzzy thinking, let alone how to reverse it! But we definitely can and it is so worth it. Eighty-six percent of people who took the ATP reported that the strategies for rebalancing the circadian rhythm and optimizing sleep in this program helped them feel better.

Light Therapy

Since the circadian rhythm is highly dependent on light, some of the most effective ways to restore balance involve regular exposure to sunlight during the day and limiting light at night.

Bright light in the morning

A high dose of bright light first thing in the morning, usually within the first hour of waking, helps us to have that beautiful high cortisol release to kick-start our day (known as the cortisol awakening response). Natural sunlight is the best source of bright light and it contains the full spectrum of colors and wavelengths of lights (like a rainbow). It is rich in blue light, a short-wavelength light that sends a strong signal to the brain that it's time to be awake, boosting attention, reaction times, and mood. Studies have found that exposure to short-wavelength light in the morning significantly enhances the cortisol awakening response compared to dim light.

Wise mothers know that getting lots of bright light in the morning also helps their young children sleep better. If the weather permits, try to get yourself outside as soon as you wake up. Yes, it's possible even if you are a parent. Some parents love early-morning stroller walks. I like having coffee or tea on the patio while my son plays nearby. Even a few minutes a day can help. If you don't live in a perpetually sunny place, there's still hope. I know getting morning sun can be tough in northern climates, especially in the winter, so using devices such as a light therapy or a blue-light lamp (also known as a "happy" or SAD [seasonal affective disorder] therapy lamp) in the morning and blue-light-blocking glasses at night can help mimic these natural cycles. Recent studies suggest that blue-light therapy may boost immune cell function, and blue-light-therapy devices have also been studied in SAD, a.k.a. "the winter blues," with great success.

For me, getting morning sun when it's sunny and using my light therapy lamp when it's not have been critical for healing my circadian rhythm, reversing morning fatigue, and boosting my cortisol levels.

I personally struggled with seasonal affective disorder for most of my life, until I moved to Southern California, when the seasonal affective disorder vanished. I didn't think much of it, until it came back when I moved back to Chicago in 2011. This particular winter was so cold, long, and gloomy that Chicago was nicknamed "Chi-beria" (get it? like Siberia). I left California optimistic and happy in January, but by March I found myself sad and tearful. The light therapy box helped my mood and energy levels significantly within a few short days, and I used it every winter while in Chicago, some days in sunny but snowy Colorado, and most days while living in romantic, rainy Amsterdam! It can also be really helpful if you have trouble waking up in the morning. I recommend keeping a blue light at your bedside and turning it on when you wake up, or keeping it in your bathroom and turning it on while you get ready.

Natural sunlight throughout the day

Through light receptors at the back of our eyes, the brain registers the changing intensity of natural sunlight throughout the day to know where it is in the twenty-four-hour cycle and sync up bodily functions (and cortisol release) accordingly.

Limit artificial light at night

Blue light sends a strong signal to the brain that it's time to be awake, increasing cortisol and boosting attention, reaction times, and mood. This is helpful when we want to make more cortisol in the morning and during the day, but it can become disruptive if we're exposed to it at night, when we're trying to wind down. Many of us have trouble sleeping and produce excess cortisol at the wrong times simply because of the blue light emitted from LED lightbulbs and televisions, computers, and smartphone screens too late in the day. All of that blue light is telling the brain it's daytime when we just want to go to sleep already! Later in the day and evening we want to limit our exposure to blue light and signal the brain that it's time to prepare for rest.

LIGHT AND THE CIRCADIAN RHYTHM

Even though we're bathed in light 24/7, many of us aren't getting enough of the right kind of light to support circadian rhythm balance and the optimal release of cortisol. While lightbulbs are great for helping us see, they're not so great when it comes to helping us sync up to the natural rise and fall of light over the course of a twenty-four-hour day.

Not only does the intensity of the artificial lights that illuminate our homes and offices remain static throughout the day, making it hard for the brain to register changes and the passing of time, artificial lights are much less intense than natural outdoor sunlight.

A well-lit indoor room may expose our eyes to anywhere from 100 to 500 lux of light (a standard measurement of how much light reaches an object—or retina!—roughly three feet away from the light source). Yet, outside on a bright, cloudless day we could be exposed to up to 150,000 lux. Even a cloudy day could expose us to 1,000 lux! The intensity of natural sunlight gets us much closer to the estimated 10,000 lux the brain needs to trigger the cortisol awakening response, and the wavelength of the light it provides also matters.

When thinking about light and the circadian rhythm, I find it helpful to give it the "caveperson test" and consider: Would ancient people have been exposed to light at this time? Living in sync with day and night was a lot simpler without streetlamps, email, indoor jobs, and streaming television! But by implementing the simple eating and lifestyle strategies included in the ATP, we can restore balance.

Light Modifications for Cortisol Levels

If you are experiencing . . .

Low Cortisol	Cortisol Roller Coaster	High Cortisol
Prioritize getting bright light in the morning and afternoon to boost cortisol naturally.	Prioritize both getting bright light in the morning and afternoon and blocking bright lights and blue lights after sunset.	Prioritize blocking bright lights and blue lights after sunset to prevent an increase in cortisol in the evening.

Daily Habits

We can use other daily habits to consistently tell the body when it should be awake and when it should rest.

Find your sleep window

Though it varies from person to person, we all have a window of time when we grow tired and ready for sleep. If we stay up too late and miss that window, we risk getting a cortisol-driven "second wind" that can keep us awake for hours. For many people, this window is between 9 and 11 p.m., though it does change with the seasons, growing later as the sun sets later.

Develop a bedtime routine

Our minds and bodies love consistency. When we create a routine around going to bed, such as taking an Epsom salt bath or listening to relaxing music, our minds recognize that it's time to lower cortisol, relax, and enter restoration mode.

Keep your sleep space cool, dark, and soothing, like a cave!

Sleeping in a space that is dark, cool, and quiet will help you sleep better and wake up feeling more rested. Your body temperature falls naturally at night, and sleeping in a cooler environment (between 60 and 67 degrees Fahrenheit) allows your body to sleep deeper and cycle through its sleep stages and, in my experience, it can also resolve nightmares. Try lowering your thermostat (or opening a window) or promoting optimal core-body temperature with a cooling mattress pad like the ChiliSleep Chilipad. Use a white/pink noise machine to block outside sounds. I personally like to use an air purifier that not only makes the air clean in my room but also makes white noise (my favorite is the AirDoctor). The Hatch Rest is an option for a stand-alone sound machine that has a variety of sounds you may enjoy. Where possible, use bedding with natural materials that are free from harmful substances like polybrominated diphenyl ethers (PBDEs). Last, but not least, make sure the room is pitch-black to optimize your melatonin production. When even a little bit of light is present, melatonin production drops and sleep can be disrupted. You may benefit from using blackout curtains or blinds, turning off all gadgets in your bedroom, and/or putting dark-colored stickers/tape over the lights emitted from the devices in your bedroom.

Start an evening-time journaling habit

Oftentimes, the inability to fall asleep stems from the stress of an overactive mind spiking cortisol. When we are worried about all of the things on our to-do list for tomorrow, or when we keep replaying the argument we had with our spouse earlier that day, it becomes nearly impossible to stop the thought cycle and fall asleep. Sometimes, just the act of writing down the thoughts that are on our minds can ease the hold they have over us and allow us to let go and rest.

Use lavender essential oil

Some individuals with adrenal issues have a surge of cortisol right before bed, known as the "second wind," that prevents them from being able to fall asleep even when they're tired. Lavender essential oil can be used to promote a calm and restful sleep. Popular ways to use it include: in a bedside diffuser, placing a few drops of the oil on your pillow, or diluting the essential oil in a carrier oil like coconut oil for topical application on the skin.

Adjust your exercise

Intense exercise can raise cortisol levels immediately afterward, which can interfere with sleep. Try to exercise no later than two hours prior to your bedtime. If you love to exercise in the evenings, consider low-intensity, sleep-promoting exercises such as restorative yoga (a restful practice where poses are held for longer), stretching, and tai chi.

Move your caffeine earlier

I mentioned that caffeine is a consequence and exacerbating factor in adrenal function. Caffeine intake can lead to trouble sleeping by elevating cortisol levels. A 2013 study found that drinking caffeinated beverages at bedtime, three hours before bed, and even six hours before bed can affect sleep. A good rule of thumb: Generally, don't have coffee less than eight hours before bedtime. See What About Caffeine? on p. 157 for guidance on how to adjust your caffeine intake.

Consider relaxing beverages at bedtime

Herbal teas, including chamomile, catnip, passionflower, and tulsi tea, can help promote restful sleep. See Balancing Teas on page 161 for more information on the benefits and precautions of various teas. The adaptogenic mushroom reishi is also calming. I like sipping on Four Sigmatic Mushroom Hot Cacao Mix with Reishi.

TRACK YOUR SLEEP

I encourage you to track your sleep during the program. You can get really fancy with devices and apps (I like the Oura Ring) or use your health journal to note the time you went to bed, the time you woke up, and the quality of your sleep. Pay attention to how different lifestyle changes, foods, and supplements impact your sleep. Not every person is the same, and some cues to signal the body that it's time to wake or sleep may be more effective for you than for others.

Circadian Timing of Foods and Supplements

We know that the adrenals are tied to the circadian rhythm and sleep deprivation is the fastest way to get into adrenal dysfunction. In order to set the stage for more energy during the day and better sleep at night, we can leverage the power of circadian nutrition. Just like sleeping and waking, digestion is tied to the circadian rhythm and by eating our meals and certain foods and supplements in alignment with it, we can set the stage for more energy during the day and better sleep at night. Consuming the right foods and beverages at the right time helps support a healthy cortisol curve.

We already talked about moving caffeine to earlier in the day and utilizing herbal teas and adaptogens to help balance the daily rhythm (page 157), and you are already practicing circadian nutrition by balancing your blood sugar. Blood sugar swings can lead to cortisol dips during the day and cortisol surges in the middle of the night. If you've ever woken up around 2 or 3 a.m. with anxious thoughts and needed a snack to fall back to sleep, that's a sign that your blood sugar needs balancing.

Another way to support circadian rhythm balance is to eat when the sun is out (preferably in a well-lit area, optimally outside) and to avoid eating after the sun sets (this shortened eating window is sometimes known as intermittent fasting).

You can get started with eating lots of food during the day and outside right away—the ATP diet schedule is set up for this. We'll eat the majority of our calories earlier in the day, starting off with a substantial breakfast (a giant smoothie!) followed by a big salad or soup for lunch. We'll taper off in the evening with a smaller meal for dinner of vegetables and protein.

However, in the initial stages of balancing your blood sugar, you may need to eat frequently and even snack right before bed and that's okay. As your blood sugar balance progresses, you may be able to partake in intermittent fasting.

In the meantime, there are other eating strategies we can implement:

- Eating a high-fat diet in the morning ensures that the body has enough cholesterol and fatty acids to produce hormones and energy when they are needed most. The Adrenal Kick Start (page 297) followed by a green smoothie (like my Root Cause Green Smoothie on page 304) about one hour later fits the bill! Eating grapefruit in the morning (but not in the evening) can also slow down the breakdown of cortisol. Grapefruit has a lot of drug interactions, so please be sure to check with your pharmacist if you take any medications.
- Energy-boosting adaptogens and B vitamins are best taken in the morning so that they can help you make more energy when you need it and not keep you buzzing all night.

- Licorice (contained in Rootcology Adrenal Support) or used as a stand-alone supplement is also best taken in the morning to help stretch the morning cortisol.
- The Maca Latte (page 300) with good fat and adaptogenic maca or the Tulsi Tea Latte (page 302) can be used in the morning and to counteract an afternoon energy dip.
- Magnesium and myo-inositol both have sleep-promoting effects and are best used at bedtime.
- Eating omega-3-rich fish at dinner can help with reducing cortisol levels to promote rest and relaxation.

....

As your circadian rhythm rebalances with these lifestyle changes, you should soon be having an easier time falling and staying asleep, as well as feeling more refreshed and energetic throughout the day. If your sleep continues to be an issue, please know that we will revisit sleep issues later on in the program and do a deeper dive, if necessary, to identify some of the other factors that could be contributing to your trouble sleeping and discuss advanced strategies to address them.

Action Steps
To reenergize, aim to:
- Drink a sufficient number of ounces of water per day based on your weight and make sure to replenish electrolytes through electrolyte-rich foods, high-quality sea salt, hydration blends, and/or an electrolyte blend supplement.
- Love your mitochondria! Consider a carnitine supplement for extra support.
- Get bright light in the morning, plenty of natural light during the day, limit artificial light at night, and time other daily habits to rebalance the circadian rhythm and improve sleep, energy, and mood, and restore hormone balance.

To view the scientific references cited in this chapter, please visit us online at https://thyroidpharmacist.com/atpbooknotes.

CHAPTER **6**

Revitalize

Goals

- Let your body know it's safe through positive thoughts and pleasurable activities.
- Treat yourself with extra love and compassion each day.
- Swap your inner critic for an encouraging friend and ally.

Our bodies need to feel safe in order to feel good, and when they feel good, they feel safe. Under threat, our bodies shift from rest, digest, and healing mode into a state of chronic stress that ramps up our fight-or-flight response and pushes our HPA axis to its limit. The key to restoring health is to send the body messages of safety so it knows that it can switch off survival mode and focus on healing. We've already explored six powerful safety signals that can be sent with diet, supportive supplements, and lifestyle. This chapter is all about how being good to ourselves can help us revitalize and recover—and reignite our joie de vivre.

Unfortunately, we can't just tell our bodies directly, "Hey, we're safe now. Time to heal!" We have to speak to them in a language they understand and send safety signals through our mindset and actions. In this chapter, we'll use positive thought patterns, self-compassion, pleasurable activities, and simple acts of self-expression to send safety signals that shift us into a healing, parasympathetic state that has been shown to relieve stress and anxiety, fight inflammation, support the immune system, boost mood, and lift libido.

1. **Positive thought patterns:** A large part of healing is having a positive mindset. We'll choose to send ourselves positive, healing messages to shift our bodies from flight-or-flight mode into "rest and digest" mode and provide an extra dose of confidence and motivation to achieve our health and life goals.

2. **Pleasurable activities:** Doing what makes us feel good prompts the release of the "love" hormone oxytocin—a simple but super-powerful way to de-stress!

3. **Creating just because:** Doodling, knitting, scrapbooking, finger painting, or making absolutely *anything* promotes calm and a positive mindset. We'll let our imaginations run free to find ways of expressing ourselves.

For many of my clients, these "prescriptions" are the most transformative of the ATP. As Diana S. shared: "Most/many of my symptoms are resolved. [Most helpful have been] the behavioral parts: setting up better daily routines, allowing more time for sleep and relaxation." I hope they bring you better health, less stress, and more joy, too!

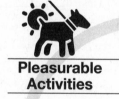

Pleasurable Activities

Positive Thought Patterns

Revitalize

Creating Just Because

Safety Signal #1: Positive Thought Patterns

"Whether you think you can or can't, you are right."—attributed to
Henry Ford

Did you know research has shown that negative thoughts can cause inflammation in our bodies? It's only natural that having numerous stress symptoms can make a person feel like a powerless victim. But when we are in a defeatist victim state, we give away our power and get stuck in negative thought patterns that alert our body that we are not safe and there's no use trying to get better.

Most important, these thought patterns prevent us from realizing just how powerful we are. I know this, because I've been there. I used to believe that I was a victim to life's circumstances and felt there was no use in trying to change my life.

I didn't think I could heal (because the doctors told me that Hashimoto's was incurable) and I thought I would be stuck with my symptoms forever. I felt so powerless. But we always have the power to make a choice. We can choose to stay in a victim mentality and wait for someone to save us, or we can take on an empowered, positive, and healing mindset and be our own savior. I began to transform my life by looking in my mirror and saying, "I am Izabella Wentz. I am in charge of my own destiny."

The late Louise Hay, the legendary founder of Hay House and author of *You Can Heal Your Life*, believed that the thoughts we think and the words we speak create our experiences and play an important role in our health. She found that specific thought patterns were tied to specific conditions and symptoms.

I was intrigued with her work when she mentioned that being stuck in a thought pattern of humiliation, having an inability to express our creative energy, and feeling like we never get to do what we want to do contribute to thyroid dysfunction. People with these patterns may feel like they spend their whole lives pleasing others and that they live their whole lives for others. (This can include fathers, mothers, bosses, spouses/lovers, children, etc.)

The thought patterns she noted in people with adrenal issues were defeatism, no longer caring for the self, severe emotional malnutrition, and anger at the self. The thought patterns in those with anxiety and insomnia were not trusting the flow and process of life, while those with fatigue were associated with resistance, boredom, and lack of love for what one does. Additionally, the symptom of low blood pressure, commonly seen in adrenal dysfunction, was also tied to defeatism, as well as lack of love as a child. Do any of these patterns resonate with you? List them below:

1.
2.
3.

But just as negative thought patterns can contribute to disease, positive thought patterns can help with creating health.

Émile Coué was a French pharmacist and psychologist who found that positive thoughts could improve healing. Positive thoughts can come in the form of affirmations, which you can repeat throughout the day. Émile Coué's original affirmation is actually one of my favorite ones, and what I used on my Hashimoto's healing journey: "Every day in every way I am getting better and better." Using affirmations, we can break the cycle of negativity and support our transformation.

Repeating these positive statements throughout the day helps repattern your thinking, uplift your outlook, and lessen the effects of stress. Some additional affirmations I've found helpful include:

- I love myself.
- I am powerful.
- I am healing.
- I am loved.
- The world is a safe and beautiful place.
- I am beautiful.

Additionally, here are some affirmations that my program participants have shared:

- I'm in charge of how I feel and I choose happiness.
- I release negative feelings and thoughts about myself.

- I don't sweat the small stuff.
- I am worthy!
- I am safe and I am protected.
- I am resilient!
- I can do hard things!
- Every day in every way I am getting better and better!
- I am a strong person; I conquer anything I put my mind to.

AFFIRMATIONS FOR SPECIFIC SYMPTOMS

Louise Hay has taken this work deeper by recommending that we identify our current thought patterns and embrace a new thought pattern utilizing affirmations tailored to each condition.

Louise Hay's Affirmations for Specific Symptoms

Hypothyroidism: I move beyond old limitations and now allow myself to express myself freely and creatively.

Adrenal issues: I love and approve of myself. It is safe for me to care for myself; I lovingly take care of my body, my mind, and my emotions.

Anxiety: I love and approve of myself and I trust the process of life. I am safe.

Low blood pressure: I now choose to live in the ever-joyous NOW. My life is a joy.

Fatigue: I am enthusiastic about life and filled with energy and enthusiasm.

Insomnia: I lovingly release the day and slip into peaceful sleep, knowing tomorrow will take care of itself.

Menstrual problems: I accept my full power as a woman and accept all my bodily processes as normal and natural. I love and approve of myself.

Below, I invite you to write some healing affirmations that you would like to incorporate throughout the ATP and beyond. Feel free to use the ones above or make up your own. You can visit this page often to not only review, but also to add to the list whenever you feel the need to do so. You may also want to take a photo of this page with your smartphone so you can refer to it on the go.

_____

_____

_____

_____

_____

_____

_____

_____

Affirmations are a form of self-compassion, and being kind to ourselves yields real physical and mental health benefits. Kristin Neff, PhD, a leading researcher on self-compassion, has found that self-kindness leads to many rewards, including increased happiness, optimism, personal initiative, and reduced anxiety. People who practice self-compassion, according to Neff, are less likely to be critical of themselves and anxious or depressed, leading to a greater capacity to make meaningful changes in their lives and greater life satisfaction. Other research has shown similar results, connecting those who are self-compassionate with less anxiety, depression, and fear of failure.

In one study, students who were instructed to direct kind and compassionate thoughts to themselves had lower heart rates and a lower sweat response at the end of the experiment than those participants who were encouraged to think critically about themselves. The head researcher, Dr. Hans Kirschner, concluded, "These findings suggest that being kind to oneself switches off the threat response and puts the body in a state of safety and relaxation that is important for regeneration and healing."

If you are someone who is always hard on yourself and struggles with self-compassion, it may help to simply pause and think about how you would treat a sweet little child, beloved pet, or a best friend if he/she failed at something.

My clients who have practiced this have shared results similar to Dr. Kirschner's findings:

> "One lasting effect of the program that was very helpful is that the spiral of negative self-talk has gotten so much easier to stop!! And reprogramming how I talk to myself has been a *huge* help. This program was very helpful in more than just healing from an ailment. It helped me hold more compassion for myself and really helped me stop the cycle of negativity toward myself."—Ludmila

Now that we know how to use our thought patterns and self-talk to support healing, let's discover how to show ourselves kindness and gentleness through our actions. You are worth it!

Safety Signal #2: Pleasurable Activities

Many of us are juggling multiple responsibilities and demands on our attention and time, often looking after both children and elderly parents (known as the sandwich generation). There is too little time to sleep, let alone meet up with friends, pursue a hobby, or have "me" time. Self-care is put on the back burner. But, as therapist Laura Koziej, MA, LCPC, has noted, this can lead to burnout, depression, and anxiety and have significant physical consequences, "such as a weaker immune system, strain on the heart, and obesity due to not having the energy to exercise and eat healthy meals." It's understandable that we want to make sure the people we love have everything they need to thrive, but in order to be able to care for others, we need to care for ourselves. Allocating time for self-care is a way of making sure we have the energy and focus to be present in all of the ways that matter for our loved ones. It can seem a little counterintuitive, but taking time for ourselves enables us to give more to others. By investing in self-care, you and everyone around you will feel the benefits!

What Makes You Feel Good?

When our days are interesting and include people and activities that make us happy, our entire outlook is more likely to be optimistic, which helps us manage stress. Perhaps you're enriched and enlivened by an early-morning walk through a local park, a quiet hour with a good book, a phone conversation with your sister, bedtime story hour with your kids, or a few minutes browsing your favorite local shop. No matter how brief, the moments that make us feel better throughout our days contribute, bit by bit, to a sense of safety and a positive mindset.

On the other hand, when our days are loaded with things that don't make us happy—senseless tasks, aimless meetings, frustrating people (I call these tasks "eating frogs")—we feel dull, weighed down, and easily discouraged. Our bodies are stressed out and drained of energy.

Additionally, loneliness and isolation, feelings that were quite common during the recent pandemic, can cause stress as well. You can also have feelings of loneliness even when you are around people you care about. I encourage you to make an honest assessment of how you feel about your day-to-day activities and the people you see most often, to understand where changes are possible and necessary.

Many of us know that there are things that make us feel better and things that make us feel worse. Yet we spend our days "eating the frogs," without giving ourselves an opportunity to do the things that make us feel good. My friends, let me tell you, the things that make you feel good are often the things that are healing.

If you're at a point where you're not sure about what makes you feel better, or worse, I encourage you to keep reading because this chapter is specifically designed to help you discover how to do more of what you find pleasurable and revitalizing and less of what drains you. Let's start with a simple but revolutionary exercise. I hope it gives you the permission slip you need to do more of what you love, and less of what you don't.

When I work with my clients, I have them take a sheet of paper and draw a line down the middle. On the left, they write "Makes Me Feel Better" and on the right, they write "Makes Me Feel Worse." And then I encourage them to fill in the details and we work on figuring out how to incorporate things from the Feel Good column into their daily life, and minimize the things from the Feel Worse column.

Laura P., a program participant, mentioned that by making a list of things she enjoys doing and just putting more of that into her life helps her resilience and makes her get through to "the other end" of each day. She

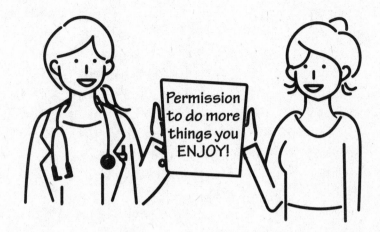

starts each morning by asking herself: "What am I gonna do that is fun today?" Doing just one small fun thing a day, even for five minutes, can make a big difference!

Makes Me Feel Better	Makes Me Feel Worse

Use the Senses to Boost Oxytocin

Our senses are always tuned in to our environment and sending messages to our bodies about what's going on and how best to adapt to the current situation. We want to use as many of our senses as possible to let the body know that it is safe. Through soothing touch, sounds, scents, and temperatures and otherwise pleasurably stimulating our senses, we can promote the release of oxytocin, a powerful safety-signaling chemical associated with encouraging trust, bonding, and relaxation.

You may have heard oxytocin referred to as a "love" hormone because of the role it plays in relationship-building, but it also has a powerful influence

Oxytocin Molecule

on our mental well-being, ability to heal, and even our ability to perceive pain and hunger.

Oxytocin

Oxytocin is a unique hormone that is produced in the hypothalamus and stored in the pituitary. It acts as a neurotransmitter, or chemical messenger, and can quickly shift the body into a parasympathetic, healing state. Traditionally, oxytocin has been associated with aiding childbirth, breastfeeding, and skin-to-skin contact with a baby. Oxytocin is released in large amounts during labor, causing uterine contractions, and during breastfeeding. Babies release oxytocin by sucking (have you ever seen how content babies are with their pacifiers?), and if a baby latches on to breastfeed, oxytocin release in the mom enables the milk to flow and helps the mother and baby bond. Mothers with high levels of oxytocin are more likely to be nurturing and affectionate with their children, frequently touching, grooming, murmuring to, and making eye contact with their babies, while babies who are exposed to more oxytocin can have improved developmental outcomes such as better socialization, appetite control, and improved gross motor skills. You don't need to be breastfeeding or birthing a baby to release oxytocin, as simple acts of caring and being cared for also release oxytocin.

It's released when people hold hands, cuddle, make love, or bond socially (talking, laughing). One study found that people in the early stages of developing a romantic relationship had higher levels of oxytocin, compared with nonattached single people, and those heightened levels lasted for at least six months.

Researchers have used oxytocin nasal sprays to promote sociability, lower anxiety, and reduce stress levels. Additionally, oxytocin has shown that it can encourage the body to heal and repair itself and can provide anti-inflammatory and pain-relieving effects by reducing pro-inflammatory cytokines and blocking pain signals while stimulating the release of the body's natural pain relievers. In addition to lessening pain during labor, recent research supports its capacity to relieve the pain associated with headaches, chronic back pain, and IBS.

I really began to appreciate this hormone after becoming a new mom. I had my son in a crib in a room where I slept, while my husband slept in a separate room due to insomnia and new mystery health challenges. At least four times each night, I would do my nighttime pilgrimage of getting up from my bed to walk across the room to my son's crib to pick him up and feed him or console him when he woke up. I was so exhausted from the night wakings and trying to get my son to sleep better that one day I decided it was enough. When Dimitry was around eight months old, instead of putting him in a crib for naps and nighttime sleep, I decided to put the mattress on the floor and safely co-sleep with him at night, and I accidentally discovered how to leverage the power of oxytocin to put myself in a more rested, happy, healing, parasympathetic state.

I got some extra sleep, and as cuddling a baby helps release oxytocin and shift into that healing state, I was surprised at how much easier it was for me to drift back to sleep and how much better I began to feel simply by sleeping with my child, despite still waking up at least four times each night. While babies are wonderful, you do not need a cute squishy baby to make oxytocin.

While much research has been done to determine how lab-made oxytocin could treat a range of conditions, there's also no need for a prescription to support your body's natural production of oxytocin. Spending time with "our people," the ones who "get" us and love us, is a great way to boost oxytocin for us extroverts, but both introverts and extroverts may want to look into other ways we can use our senses to add more oxytocin to our day-to-day life through touch, laughter, smell, sound, and warmth. I hope you will soon be eager to try at least one of these oxytocin-boosting activities and find ways to incorporate them into your routine!

Physical touch

Healing touch can quickly boost our oxytocin levels and drop our stress levels! Research has shown that the simple act of hugging can increase oxytocin levels, and if you only do one thing on this list, let it be getting more from your loved ones! Touching, cuddling, affectionate caressing, or even sitting close to someone we care about boosts oxytocin and all of its stress-relieving, bond-building positive effects. How many hugs should you aim for? Therapist Virginia Satir is credited with proposing, "We need four hugs a day for survival. We need 8 hugs a day for maintenance. We need 12 hugs a day for growth." I don't know about you, but I can definitely get behind the twelve-hugs-per-day challenge. ☺

You don't have to limit yourself to humans, either. Studies have shown oxytocin levels increase in both human and dog following a petting or stroking session, which is why you both feel better after physical contact (my dog, Boomer, and I concur). And yes, fellow cat lovers, it's true for cats, rabbits, and even non-cuddly animals like turtles. I prefer petting animals that are cuddly, but it was amazing to see how my son lit up when petting lizards and a roly-poly that we recently found in nature! And the benefits aren't limited to pet owners. When I lost a loved one to suicide, I found comfort in stopping at a pet store that was on my way home from work. There was a time when I would drop in and snuggle with the puppies and kittens most days, and I think the sweet animals benefited, too. If you don't have your own pet, offer to pet sit or visit an animal shelter. Animals need hugs just as much as we do!

If you don't have access to a real animal, I have a little secret you may have forgotten about from your childhood: Cuddling something soft, like a stuffed animal or blanket, can release oxytocin and bring us comfort as well. Yes, even if you are an adult! These days my son has a stuffed baby doll, goat, and Spider-Man that he likes to sleep with, and will sometimes ask me to hold them, and you know what? It always makes me smile! In researching this book, I was intrigued to learn that after trying to reunite over seventy-five thousand forgotten teddy bears, the hotel chain Travelodge conducted a survey that found 35 percent of British adults admitted they sleep with their teddy because they found cuddling their bear helps them to de-stress and fall asleep after a hard day.

Another option (perhaps more biohacker friendly)? A weighted blanket. Resembling a standard blanket but with beads or pellets to give them added heft, weighted blankets help relieve stress and anxiety by mimicking the sensation of a comforting hug or being "tucked in" by a loved one. I recommend using a weighted blanket that is 7 to 15 percent of your body weight and checking with your healthcare provider to make sure it's a good option for you. Weighted blankets may not be appropriate for those with sleep apnea or other sleep disorders, respiratory problems, or other chronic conditions.

But to be soothed by a hug, all you really need is you. Simply give yourself a squeeze after a rough day or when you feel dialed up. According to leading self-compassion researcher Kristin Neff, a warm, caring hug increases feelings of love and tenderness toward the self. Or, try the butterfly hug, an easy relaxation and self-soothing technique developed by therapist Lucy Artigas while assisting children and adults in the aftermath of Hurricane Pauline in Acapulco, Mexico, in 1998. Originally created to be used with eye movement desensitization and reprocessing (EMDR) therapy, a trauma-focused therapy that gives the brain novel ways to reprocess traumatic memories, the butterfly hug can be used as a stress reliever on its own. It works by activating both sides of the brain at the same time, called bilateral stimulation, and thus syncing feeling with learning to relax the body and mind. To give yourself a butterfly hug, cross your arms, place your fingers on your chest, just under the collarbone, and tap your hands left-right-left-right, like fluttering butterfly wings, for at least eight rounds, until you feel more relaxed. Try this now! I bet you will smile. ☺

One of my favorite forms of healing touch is massage therapy. After just fifteen minutes of massage, participants in a 2012 study felt more relaxed and had higher oxytocin levels. Different types of massage therapy modalities are available to suit almost anyone's need. Some examples are Swedish massage (smooth, long strokes, my favorite), hot stone massage, and reflexology (application of pressure to areas of the feet and hands). In 2015, I conducted a survey of my readers. In total, 2,232 people answered the survey, 1,991 of whom reported having Hashimoto's. Of the readers I surveyed, 62 percent found that massage therapy helped their pain. As a bonus, 80 percent found it beneficial for mood as well. Interestingly, one study asked hospitalized patients to rate their pain levels on a scale of 1 to 10, before and after receiving massage therapy. The average rating before therapy was 5.81. After therapy, it dropped to 2.33, with patients also reporting improvements in emotional well-being, relaxation, and their ability to sleep. A reputable massage therapist can help you decide which type of therapy would be most beneficial for you. If you'd rather not leave the comfort of your own home, consider an in-home, on-demand service. My favorite is Zeel. Or tap your partner for some couples massage. In one small study, couples reported their physical and emotional well-being significantly improved after a massage session with their partner, even though they lacked professional experience and training. That's the power of oxytocin in action.

Laughter Rx

Laughter truly is the best medicine and known to boost oxytocin levels, lower stress, and give your immune system a boost. Reach out to your partner or grab a friend, and do some positive bonding—but only if doing so gives you energy. While many of my clients like to reach out to loved ones and feel a sense of community when they are feeling down, others say they prefer to do some serious cocooning, hiding away and hunkering down alone. If you are energized by socializing, know that bonding with dear friends and sharing laughter can raise oxytocin levels and help counter the negative effects of our stress hormone, cortisol.

Of course, there are other ways to laugh, such as watching funny videos or movies, reading or listening to a silly book (I love Janet Evanovich), or going to a comedy show. Do whatever makes you laugh—with others or on your own!

Aromatherapy

Aromatherapy, an ancient healing modality that uses natural plant extracts to improve physical and emotional well-being, can be used to trigger relaxing and calming feelings. For more than a thousand years cultures around the world have used plants, roots, and herbs to make aromatic balms and oils for mood-enhancing, medicinal, and religious purposes. The term "aromatherapy" was first used in 1937 by René-Maurice Gattefossé, a French chemist who did much to advance our understanding of the potential therapeutic uses of essential oils. Essential oils are compounds extracted from plants via distillation or mechanical extraction, such as cold pressing, which retains the unique healing properties of each plant. These compounds contain the plants' aromas and flavors, or "essences," in an ultra-concentrated form. Today, essential oils are so popular you've probably spotted them in your local grocery store!

Much of the benefit from aromatherapy is thought to be derived from the scent of the essential oils. Scent is thought to be tied to memory (the olfactory, or "smell," system and the memory system of the brain are interconnected), and I am certain that I'm not the only person who can be impacted by a passing scent (the smell of gardenia trees always sparks joyful memories of visiting my grandmother's house in the spring, while the cologne of a deceased loved one can bring me to tears any day).

Studies have shown that inhaling essential oils can calm the mind and relax the body, leading to lowered stress levels, better sleep, and more balanced hormones, by allowing hormones to reset themselves. I was fascinated to see studies that found that clary sage and lavender could increase oxytocin levels.

There are many different ways in which essential oils can be used, including diffusing them in the air, using them topically (I always recommend putting them in a carrier oil, such as almond or coconut oil, to avoid burns and irritation to the skin), or adding them to a bath. My favorite way is soaking in a tub with Epsom salts and lavender essential oil! I do not recommend ingesting them unless you consult a knowledgeable expert trained in using essential oils internally.

Please note, certain oils are contraindicated for use around pets, pregnant women, nursing mothers, and young children. Additionally, those with multiple chemical sensitivities, salicylate reactions, and asthma may need to avoid essential oils altogether. However, most people are able to use essential oils, and for many, they have become an important part of a daily routine that has helped them overcome stress, which, in turn, has made an impact on their overall health.

I've included some of the most beneficial oils for stress relief below. I recommend starting with one or two of these, and seeing how you feel.

MY FAVORITE STRESS-RELIEVING ESSENTIAL OILS

Lavender (*Lavandula angustifolia*)
- Supports restful sleep, produces antianxiety effects, and increases oxytocin levels

Frankincense (*Boswellia carterii*, *B. frereana*, and *B. sacra*)
- Promotes feelings of calm and relaxation
- Supports the immune, nervous, and digestive systems
- May support thyroid health

Bergamot (*Citrus bergamia*)
- Dissolves anxious feelings while uplifting one's emotions
- Cleanses and purifies the mind and body

Cedarwood (*Juniperus virginiana*)
- Soothes the mind and body to promote vitality and relaxation
- Aids in emotional balance and overall wellness
- Allows the body to find a natural calm and increases confidence

Clary Sage (*Salvia sclarea*)
- Supports oxytocin, provides calm and relaxation to the mind and body
- Alleviates muscle tension and cramping
- Supports a restful night's sleep by calming mental chatter

Wild Orange (*Citrus sinensis*)
- Uplifts and energizes the mind and body
- Eases digestive discomfort

- Purifies and stimulates the body's systems, especially the immune system

When purchasing essential oils, look for:
- A tightly sealed amber- or dark-colored bottle.
- A label that lists the Latin name, "100 percent pure essential oil," and all of the ingredients. (If you are shopping for a pure essential oil, it should have only one ingredient.)
- A pleasant, crisp, and natural scent. If the scent gives you a headache or simply turns you off in some way, steer clear. If purchasing online, check reviews for any complaints.
- A reasonable cost. If the price seems too good to be true, it probably is!
- A company committed to high standards of quality control. Their website should be transparent about their quality standards and commitment to them. I suggest purchasing directly from a trusted company or a specialty or natural health store to ensure the product's authenticity.

Sound therapy

In the modern world, we are constantly bombarded with toxicity . . . and I don't just mean from pesticides and pollution.

- "This just in" cable news reports initiate our fight-or-flight response, releasing epinephrine to keep us glued to the TV, waiting for the latest updates. (How many times have you turned on CNN to hear a "breaking news" story? Epinephrine stresses our adrenals, changes our gut microbes to become more pathogenic, and can be addictive.)
- Social media algorithms keep us scrolling . . .
- Talk radio blasts out arguments and controversy . . .
- Gossip websites cry drama, drama, drama . . .

- Media companies use these strategies to pull in the largest audience and get the most money from advertisers . . .
- "Independent" email marketers use fear-based copy to generate frenzied sales . . .

Even movies and songs can set off our survival mode. Have you ever had a nightmare after a movie? Some of us may be more sensitive to different types of media. Growing up, my parents always blasted the news but got stressed out whenever my brother or I played our favorite music (gangster rap, heavy metal, and punk rock). I cannot watch negative news, horror or violent movies, but I can listen to any type of music. Meanwhile, my husband has no problem with movies but gets triggered by negative news and social media.

I recommend tuning out the negative news, music, and other media that makes you feel bad. It may not sound easy, but you'll be amazed by how impactful "unplugging" can be! Here are some suggestions for avoiding triggering content:

- Stop watching the news.
- Stop tuning in to gossip.
- Unfollow people on Facebook and other social media who trigger you.
- Stop watching violent shows and movies.
- Stop listening to music that stirs up negative emotions in you.
- Unsubscribe to fear-based email newsletters.

Instead, choose to listen to healing music on a daily basis, whether that's classical, instrumental, gospel, whatever you prefer that lifts your mood and eases your mind. I like listening to music on YouTube, Pandora, or Spotify. Here are a few of my favorites:

- Medicine for the People
- Enya
- Lullabies (they work for adults, as well as for babies!)

- "Flow state" music (music designed to boost focus)
- Wholetones music (therapeutic music composed by Michael Tyrrell at a healing frequency)

Warmth

There's something about being warm and cozy that makes us feel super safe. People with thyroid and adrenal conditions are often cold, and we may need to work on warming ourselves up to feel comfortable. Warming ourselves externally helps spare some of the work that our thyroid and adrenals need to do to increase our temperature and may be helpful in boosting our metabolism. Increasing our temperature can help with clearing out toxins, circulating lymphatics, fighting infections, and raising our oxytocin levels. Increasing our body temperature usually makes us feel better!

Try these activities to increase your temperature. Please be sure to start low and go slow (or should I say, be sure to slowly *warm up* to them). ☺ Use common sense, listen to your body, and do not overdo it!

Sit on a beach or out in the sun. Beach vacations are one of my favorite recommendations for people with thyroid or adrenal conditions. Sitting on the beach in the bright sunshine immediately puts most of us at ease and provides additional benefits, including a boost of immune-strengthening vitamin D. Even without the beach, I'm a big proponent of being out in nature and enjoying the sunlight.

WHY DO I FEEL SO GOOD AT THE BEACH?

- Sunshine helps us convert cholesterol into pregnenolone.
- Warmth boosts our oxytocin levels.
- Daytime bright lights cause our pupils to constrict, which helps to turn on the parasympathetic system.
- Sunlight increases vitamin D, an essential nutrient for the immune system and bone health and better mood.

Sauna therapy. Saunas provide many benefits, including stress relief and mood elevation. One of the main reasons they feel so good is because the heat of the sauna causes levels of beta-endorphins, powerful pain blockers, to rise while levels of stress hormones, such as cortisol, do not. Your muscles relax, allowing your body to release tension and stress. While in the sauna, your parasympathetic nervous system takes over, putting your body in a state of complete relaxation. For my favorite infrared sauna, check out Recommended Products at http://thyroidpharmacist.com/atpbookbonus.

Hot or warm yoga. Yoga is a great way to boost oxytocin, work up a sweat, release toxins, and engage in a low-impact yet challenging exercise. Additionally, the combination of physical movement with focused attention to breath involved in yoga allows you to clear your mind while strengthening your mind-body connection. Turning up the temperature during your practice turns up the benefits! Hot yoga typically means a vigorous form of yoga practiced in a heated, humid room, sometimes reaching as high as 105 degrees Fahrenheit. Bikram yoga is a particularly intense type. These classes may be too challenging for those in the later stages of adrenal dysfunction, so instead I recommend practicing out in the sunshine for added warmth and a dose of vitamin D!

Hot or warm baths with Epsom salt. I have a confession. I am a hot Epsom salt bath junkie! Taking a blissful warm bath is one of the simplest and fastest ways to get the body relaxed and full of oxytocin. The warm bath has been one of the main reasons I have been able to keep it together even after long days of pharmacy school, patient advocacy, pregnancy, parenting a toddler, and the pandemic! My husband loves them, too, and we each take turns having one-on-one time with our son while the other parent takes a bath. My hubby jokes that our daily baths are better than any kind of marriage therapy.

Adding Epsom salts, a form of magnesium, boosts magnesium levels in your body, just as taking a supplement can, helping to create a calming effect and alleviating joint and muscle pain.

I recommend using Epsom salts in place of bath bombs as the chemical dyes, fragrances, and glitter many of them contain can irritate the skin of the vagina (not fun) and disrupt the vaginal flora, increasing the risk of yeast and urinary tract infections when used in large quantities. Also, while some people may love adding their own essential oils in carrier oils (one teaspoon of oil such as coconut or almond, mixed with a few drops of essential oil) to an Epsom salt bath, I prefer using Epsom salts that already contain essential oils to avoid mistakenly adding too much oil. Essential oils can burn the sides of your bathtub, or worse, your lady (or gentleman) parts. (Once again, these are the things I learned the hard way and I'm sharing for your benefit, not to brag about my glamorous life, ha ha.)

You can overdose on Epsom salts, so be sure not to exceed two cups in a full bathtub, and follow the package instructions. You will want to soak in a tub with Epsom salts for at least twelve minutes. Use Epsom salts with pre-added essential oils and/or play relaxing music during your bath for triple or quadruple the bliss.

More ways to add warmth. Additional ways that you can increase warmth include sipping on a warm beverage, soup, or broth; cozying up under a heated blanket; or using a heating pad. I love my lavender-scented rice-filled heating pad.

Spend time in nature

Whether it's a hiking trail, the beach, your backyard, a local park, or a community garden, taking a short walk in nature is a multisensory experience that can help you release oxytocin and de-stress. Amplify the grounding properties by taking off your shoes and feeling the earth directly against your skin. If you have access to a more forested area, consider exploring it. Research has shown that people who went "forest bathing," or spent time in a forest, were able to increase their levels of oxytocin and shift into a parasympathetic state.

....

I encourage you to take every opportunity to bring more of these oxytocin-boosting activities into your daily life. A great way to be consistent about it is to build a ritual (or two!) around one or more of these activities so that they become a regular part of your everyday, weekly, or monthly routine.

THE ATP MODALITIES I USED TO HEAL
AS A NURSING MOM

Rebalancing my adrenals as a new mom was a process. While I was already eating an anti-inflammatory, blood sugar–balanced diet and taking the probiotic *Saccharomyces boulardii* when I discovered that I had flatlined adrenals due to sleep deprivation, I couldn't rely on my usual protocols. I did many of the things I am describing in this book.

I leveraged the power of oxytocin by co-sleeping with my son (see page 187) and adding more simple, pleasurable activities to my routine, such as Epsom salt baths, smelling essential oils, and fun age-appropriate mommy and baby classes—from art to yoga—where I got to bond and socialize with other moms and sometimes even did a few yoga moves.

I focused on circadian balance by utilizing lots of outdoor time during the day. When my son was a toddler and we lived in Colorado, we spent many days at a local hiking trail and our favorite little lake. After moving to Los Angeles, we went to the beach and a local park. On days that were tough due to the fear around the pandemic or the usual mommy sleep deprivation, we often did a session of "naked baby running on the beach," where we would take our son and let him roam the beach with just his diaper or undies. It was a wonderful way to ease the stress, get vitamin D levels up, and laugh and connect as a family.

We went to bed early and slept with blackout curtains at night to boost melatonin levels. In addition to protecting mitochondria, melatonin promotes sleepiness and is released in response to darkness.

When I first discovered that my adrenals were flatlined, I was nursing a baby, so I didn't feel comfortable taking hormones and adrenal supplement blends. Some women take oral progesterone, but it seemed to drop my milk supply. Instead, I opted for holy basil (tulsi) tea. This tasty tea has adaptogenic properties and has been used as an herbal galactagogue (an herb used to promote lactation) in traditional medicine.

When my son became a little older, I incorporated carnitine, magnesium, myo-inositol, and electrolytes with the approval of his pediatrician. Carnitine can be deficient in postpartum women and was super helpful for my brain function, energy levels, and the regaining of my strength. Magnesium helped with nursing aversion and feeling more calm, while myo-inositol made me feel less anxious. For brain fog, I added additional brain-restoring supplements (choline, benfotiamine, riboflavin, and fish oil) that are generally safe and potentially beneficial in lactation. When my son was less dependent on breast milk, I added topical progesterone (see Female Hormone Imbalance in the Advanced Stress Symptom Formulary [page 348]).

I had already been on a personal growth journey and had done lots of EMDR prior to my son's birth, but did not have much time for additional deep work. Instead, I focused on using the NeurOptimal neurofeedback machine to help my brain be more calm and less reactive. I did sessions while nursing my son, holding him for his naps, or while he was asleep in his own bed.

I wasn't able to simplify my home or declutter until he got a little older, but I did seek in-home help to support me with cooking, laundry, cleaning, and the other glamorous never-ending "mommy" tasks. I stopped tolerating people who drained my energy or made me feel anxious.

I know it can be hard to find support when we need it most in those early days with baby, so I created a Nursing Mother's Formulary for helpful functional medicine strategies and supplements. You can download a free copy, along with other helpful bonuses, at http://thyroidpharmacist.com/atpbookbonus.

Safety Signal #3: Do Something Creative Just Because

Creating something "just because" can boost levels of dopamine, a feel-good neurotransmitter that is involved in energy production, mental clarity, and motivation. Without the pressure we feel when making something we have to produce, the creative process becomes relaxing. It sends a powerful safety signal to the body by rooting us in the present moment, increasing our awareness and mindfulness, and putting us in a perfect balance of sympathetic focus with parasympathetic relaxation and regeneration, known as the "flow state." Whether it's drawing, painting, sewing, writing, or baking, I encourage you to take the time to do something creative, even if your day-to-day life or work tends to be creative. You will get the most out of the experience by letting go of expectations, having fun, and enjoying the process.

You don't even have to do traditionally artistic things to gain the benefits of creating something. I didn't have time in my busy schedule to take art classes in my undergraduate studies, but my weekly three-hour synthetic chemistry lab, where I created various chemicals, served as a place to become centered and present. When I lived with my parents, baking (it reminded me of chemistry lab!) and scrapbooking were my artsy pursuits of choice, but those stopped being relaxing after I got married and began to cook every day and had tons of photo albums to make from my wedding. I started to write for de-stressing, but since becoming a professional author with deadlines and high expectations for my writing, I have switched to making art. I really enjoy the process, and even better, I am not particularly artistic, so there's no chance of me doing art for anything other than fun, thus keeping it low stress. ☺ These days, it's usually in the form of painting or drawing with my son.

I love to put up a large blank sheet of craft paper at toddler height and set out lots of different-colored paints and a variety of foam paintbrushes for us to create our own masterwork of colorful smears and splashes. We let our imaginations run free! These activities calm my mind and allow me to "stop and smell the roses" (and keep my busy toddler engaged, too). Two of my talented team members create giftable types of art: Our nutritionist, Stephanie, sews adorable aprons, and our project manager, Tina, creates beautiful cards.

If you're looking for an easy way to incorporate art into your routine, may I suggest adult coloring books? Did you know that coloring, yes, coloring a pre-printed design, has been shown to offer the same benefits as drawing? Feel free to color right in this book, or go to http://thyroidpharmacist.com/atpbookbonus to download the printable ATP journal that contains the mandala butterfly opposite and other images for you to color in.

A TRANSFORMATIONAL MANDALA BUTTERFLY FOR YOU TO COLOR

Butterflies and mandalas are well-known, powerful symbols of transformation, and mandalas are also associated with healing. Drawing (or coloring) mandalas can really help us process emotions that we're going through. Though mandala designs may vary in shape, color, and pattern, they are intended to represent completion, balance, harmony, wholeness, and the cycle of life.

Try coloring this mandala butterfly before bed, especially if your normal before-bed activity is stimulating—like watching television or browsing the internet. While you fill in each color, think of a positive thought or affirmation, and continue to repeat it to yourself until you complete the section(s) with that color.

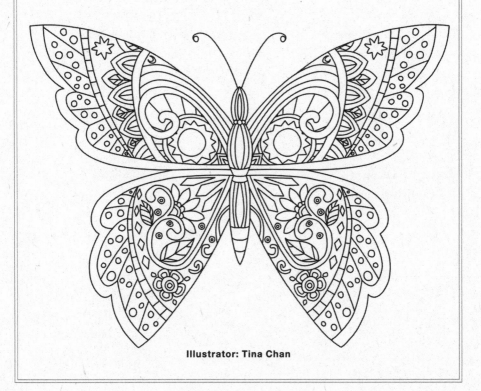

Illustrator: Tina Chan

A big thank-you to our very talented project manager, Tina, for drawing this mandala butterfly and sharing it with us!

Action Steps

To revitalize, aim to:

- Make self-compassion a priority. Start loving yourself more through words and actions today.
- Promote a positive mindset and thought patterns through affirmations.
- Crowd out what does not make you feel better with more of what does, including oxytocin-boosting practices.
- Create—just because!

To view the scientific references cited in this chapter, please visit us online at https://thyroidpharmacist.com/atpbooknotes.

CHAPTER 7

Rebuild Resilience

Goals

- Build resilience by making small changes that take you a little bit out of your comfort zone and help you become less rigid and more flexible.
- Let go of inflammatory thoughts, behaviors, and people.
- Add positive, healthy coping mechanisms and practices.
- Come to a deeper understanding of who you are as a unique individual.
- Appreciate your strengths as you discover what you need to thrive.

Why do some people break under pressure while others bend and pivot? My mentor, JJ Virgin, once said, "Don't wish it were easier. Make yourself stronger." Resilience is the key to weathering life's storms—but what is it exactly, and how do we build it?

I like to think of resilience as strength through flexibility. As Confucius wisely observed: "The green reed which bends in the wind is stronger than the mighty oak which breaks in a storm." Like the green reed, we can be at our strongest—mentally, physically, and emotionally—when we allow ourselves to change and adapt, bending old rules about who we are or how we should act and discovering new ones that suit us better. The mighty oak, strong in appearance, is fragile and vulnerable because of its rigidity. Many of us become rigid and inflexible in order to hide our own fragility and vulnerability, but in order to transform from surviving to thriving, we should aim to bring more flexibility into our lives. Otherwise, we are destined to repeat the same patterns that got us stuck in adrenal dysfunction in the first place!

In this chapter, we'll tap into some powerful healing modalities that send the body safety signals by fostering resilience. Don't worry, there's nothing extreme here. We'll skip the cold plunges and sprint intervals! ☺ Instead, we'll make small changes that take us just a little bit out of our comfort zone and focus on energizing movement, slowing down our breath, creating healthy coping strategies, letting go of the heaviness that weighs us down, and reclaiming our space.

I will introduce you to healing modalities focused on the mind and body connection that send additional safety signals through building resilience and further reducing inflammation, a top four adrenal stressor, that can leave us stiff in body and mind.

1. **Movement that makes you feel good:** Exercising in a way that invigorates rather than drains us mitigates the negative effects of chronic stress.

2. **Slowing your breath:** Breathing more slowly calms the stress response.

3. **Creating healthy coping strategies:** We can diffuse the power that triggers have over us, regain our equilibrium, and support lasting healing by choosing coping mechanisms that work for us, not against us.

4. **Letting go of the heaviness that weighs you down:** While research confirms that self-compassion is one of the most powerful ways to build resilience, survive, and thrive, sometimes that alone is not enough to drive big changes. As we practice self-compassion, we also need to identify and actively remove (perceived) barriers and inflammatory elements such as resentments, energy-sapping situations, limiting beliefs, and trauma that are blocking us from healing. As we do this, we create space to achieve our health and life goals.

5. **Reclaiming your space:** Setting boundaries is a skill we can learn—it gets easier with practice!—to limit our exposure to stress while being honest about what we expect from others and what they can expect from us.

I became a student of personal growth at the very young age of twenty-one, when I lost a loved one to suicide, and I've come to know the value of growing and changing on my own healing journey. I've also watched as many clients and community members have not only turned the corner on their symptoms but also transformed every aspect of their lives by clearing out what's no longer serving them. When inflammatory thoughts and people take up space in our lives, we are left with less room to grow and bend. I truly believe we need to clear them out so we have the space to be as flexible and strong as a reed in the wind. I hope that you, too, will experience plenty of healing through building resilience.

ATP SUCCESS STORIES

"My personal understanding of myself has improved. I didn't realize the gravity of the emotional component. I put a lot of work into those exercises and I understand the role my emotions have played in my health journey. I have been trying to protect myself by concealing a personal and emotional trauma from myself for almost 35 years now and this program forced me to face it and to start dealing with it. It's not pretty but I can handle it now. . . . You have given me tools to truly create a symptom-free life and that has helped save my life."—JACQUELYN B.

"This particular piece of the program . . . clarified particular behavior patterns and relationship patterns. It gave me knowledge and allowed me to confront what is. . . . I could see which behavior is mine and which is not. . . . That was very, very powerful and helped me to come out healthier and feel relieved. It freed up a lot of energy for me to work on my health, rather than fix those people who were bringing unhealthy behaviors into my life."—TANYA V.

"[This program is] life changing. Positive thinking, forgiveness, supplements. So many things helped me overall and then my family felt my change and their personality changed!! I'm so very thankful for this program. You have changed our lives!!!! Much love."—MARZENA

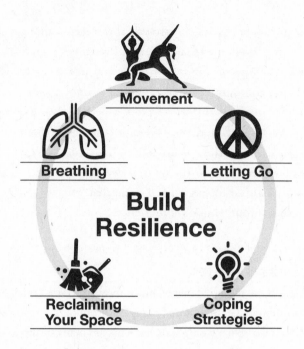

Safety Signal #1: Movement That Makes You Feel Good

Did you know that the key to whether you're doing the right exercise for the current health of your body is that you should feel better after exercising? After an exercise session, if you can't say that you could do that whole session again, right now, there's a chance that you did the wrong type of exercise, too much exercise, or both. We know that movement can help our bodies heal, but in times of adrenal stress, the wrong type of movement can be overwhelming and actually deepen our adrenal dysfunction. Many people with adrenal issues report pain, difficulty with building muscle, and feeling worse after exercise. This is because in adrenal dysfunction the body is in a catabolic state, a state of breaking itself down. To balance that, we need anabolic exercises, or exercises that build the body back up. Those will depend on your specific needs and your current stage of adrenal dysfunction. The more advanced the stage, the less likely it is that you'll be able to tolerate any type of high-intensity exercise.

If you are in Stage I or Stage II of adrenal dysfunction, you may feel on edge, rushed, and wired because cortisol is either consistently high or spiking at the wrong times. In these earlier stages, regular aerobic exercise like biking or running—at a level that you are comfortable with—can be immensely helpful because when we raise our heart rate, our bodies use up the extra circling cortisol to accelerate the breakdown of glucose, fat, and muscle protein. So in simple terms, aerobic exercise can normalize elevated cortisol, making us feel calmer and more relaxed.

But here's the thing. Heart rate–raising aerobic exercises encourage the breakdown of muscle (they are sometimes called "catabolic" exercises for this reason, in contrast to "anabolic" exercises, which build muscle). Aerobic exercise is beneficial—as long as the body has the resources to build the muscles back up stronger. Studies show that over time, regular aerobic exercise promotes muscle repair, recovery, and growth, and can help lower cortisol levels.

In people with Stage III of adrenal dysfunction, however, aerobic, catabolic activities may actually worsen the state of our muscles, as the body is already under-resourced and depleted, so it can't build them up efficiently.

An important clue as to whether we're strong enough to repair our muscles after catabolic exercise is to see how we feel after this type of exercise. Generally speaking, if you feel calmer and more relaxed after aerobic exercise, keep doing it. If you feel more tired after aerobic exercise, that's a sign that it's likely too intense and catabolic for you at this stage.

At the advanced Stage III, where total cortisol is low all day, every day, aerobic exercise can worsen this state and further reduce cortisol levels— definitely not what we want! Further lowering cortisol can lead to a hormonal cascade that lowers the amounts of other hormones known to have anabolic effects, including DHEA and testosterone (these steroids are often exploited by body builders, but our body creates them naturally). When we combine catabolic exercise with low cortisol, our muscles and the body become more broken down instead of becoming stronger. That's why a person with Stage III dysfunction may need to focus on gentle strength-training (anabolic) exercise like yoga and stretching, refuel the body with muscle-rebuilding nutrients (protein, electrolytes with ribose, and mitochondrial support are key factors), and then slowly add in more intensive muscle-building exercises, like weight lifting or Pilates, to gradually shift the body into an overall anabolic/healing state.

CATABOLIC EXERCISE

- Breaks down muscle.
- Also known as aerobic or cardio exercises.
- Less intense examples include gardening, light walking, and swimming.
- More intense forms include aerobics, running, and biking, and other activities where you maintain a steady active state for an extended period.
- People with Stage I (High Cortisol) adrenal dysfunction will feel more relaxed and calm after doing them.
- People with Stage II (Cortisol Roller Coaster) may feel better or worse depending on the time of day the exercise is done and their cortisol levels at that time.
- People with Stage III (Low Cortisol) adrenal dysfunction may consider reducing or stopping catabolic exercise during the four-week program, then gradually adding them back in as healing occurs.

ANABOLIC EXERCISE

- Builds and maintains muscle.
- Strength-training exercises.
- Gentle options include restorative, hatha, and yin yoga and stretching.
- More intensive ones include vinyasa, Ashtanga, and power yoga; weight lifting; and Pilates.
- Helpful for any stage of adrenal dysfunction, but especially important for Stage III, so long as it is an appropriate level and you are not feeling exhausted.
- A good place to start is two fifteen- to thirty-minute sessions each week, with ample time between them to recover.

Keep in mind: For some people with advanced adrenal dysfunction and deficiencies, even yoga and walking can be too much. Give one or

> more of these gentle exercise activities a try, and as always, listen to your body to determine if they are right for you.

If you're concerned that you will "balloon up" without aerobic exercise, as one of my clients said, fear not! I encourage you to try doing less than what you normally do for just a few weeks and see how you feel. One of my clients with advanced adrenal issues was surprised when I told her to stop her daily power walks, but she lost those few final stubborn pounds within a couple of weeks! This happened because rest allowed her body to switch into a more anabolic state. When we have low cortisol and overexercise, our bodies can get the message that they are not safe and respond by holding on to weight. It seems counterintuitive, but in this stage, exercising less may bring us the adrenal healing and weight loss we're looking for.

If you have low cortisol, I am not suggesting that you swear off aerobic exercise forever—it has a lot of proven benefits when done at the right time—but you will benefit from pausing aerobic exercise until your cortisol levels normalize. For some this can happen in four weeks; for others, it may take as long as two years. Please listen to your body. As you heal, you can focus on how your body responds to gentle or lighter exercise. If weight is a concern, please note that over time, an abundance of nutrients, circadian balance, and gentle and appropriate strength training can help you build muscle that will help you burn more calories and reach your goal weight.

It's important to note that exercise intolerance is also a symptom of poor mitochondrial function, a potential root cause, an exacerbating factor, or even a consequence of adrenal dysfunction. As part of nourishing and replenishing our bodies during the four-week ATP, we focus on mitochondrial-supporting nutrients available to us through foods and supplements, including B vitamins, vitamin C, magnesium, adaptogens, carnitine, and D-ribose.

The key takeaways on exercise:

1. The more cortisol you have, the more aerobic (catabolic) exercise you'll be able to tolerate. In the early stage of adrenal dysfunction when

cortisol is generally higher or spiking, aerobic exercise can help by lowering cortisol, thus bringing the body into balance.

2. In more advanced stages of adrenal dysfunction, aerobic exercise can further lower cortisol, making us feel worse.

3. Anabolic exercises, like strength training and relaxing exercises like yoga, are useful at any phase, so long as they are done at a level that does not feel tiring.

4. Exercise should be treated like a supplement or drug with each person's "prescription" completely individualized: the right exercise for them, for the right amount of time (or at the right time of day), in the right dosage (amount).

5. Check in with yourself regularly as you go, and ask: *Do I feel more relaxed or more exhausted after exercising?*

If you feel more relaxed, you've found the right exercise for your body, at the right time, in the right amount.

If you feel more exhausted, give yourself time to recuperate. Try choosing an exercise with lower intensity and/or exercising for shorter periods of time.

YOGA FOR RESILIENCE IN BODY AND MIND

We talked about utilizing yoga as a pleasurable activity in Chapter 5. I personally love outdoor yoga on sunny days, as well as hot yoga, and there are many additional types of yoga that are not just pleasurable but can also help you build resilience. In yoga, we nudge our bodies to do something that's just a little out of our comfort zone to build resilience, flexibility, and physical as well as mental strength. We focus on our breathing to stay present and calm during hard poses, and with enough experience in the yoga studio, we eventually learn to breathe and stay calm and present when we encounter hard things in life outside the yoga studio.

Safety Signal #2: Slow Your Breath to Retrain Your Brain and Body

The body is an amazing feedback machine. We tend to breathe very quickly when we are stressed. This in turn speeds up our heart rate and shifts the body into a sympathetic state. Slowing down our breath can shift us into a healing, parasympathetic state. I am always amazed at the wisdom of our ancestors. Scientists have found that yoga mantras and reciting the rosary can shift our breathing to six breaths a minute, which enhances heart rate variability, a measure of our autonomic nervous system. You can slow your breathing through ancient modalities such as prayer, yoga mantras, and meditation, as well as modern-day biofeedback and neurofeedback.

Prayer

Prayer elicits the "relaxation response," a term coined by Dr. Herbert Benson, professor, author, cardiologist, and founder of Harvard's Benson-Henry Institute for Mind Body Medicine, to describe the opposite of fight-or-flight. Prayer also promotes a sense of meaning, connection, and peace that can help you find calm, a sense of purpose, and an opportunity for self-reflection.

Yoga Mantras

Traditional yoga mantras are words that are chanted aloud or repeated in our minds that are believed to have transformative powers for mind, body, and spirit, in part by silencing mind chatter and helping us be fully aware and present. "Om" and "Om shanti" (peace) are two popular ones.

Meditation

The practice of meditation can be dated back to as early as 3000 B.C.E. in India. It involves practicing being in the present moment without expectations—this can be done while lying in silence, sitting in a park, or even walking.

Studies have found that meditation has the ability to boost levels of key hormones and neurotransmitters, including serotonin (the "happy" hormone involved in mood regulation), the calming neurotransmitter GABA, the adrenal hormone DHEA (also known as the "youth hormone"), growth hormone (helps with staying fit and muscular), and melatonin (helps with falling asleep), making meditation a particularly powerful tool for improving overall health. Research has also shown that meditation can help your adrenal glands by significantly lowering elevated cortisol levels and decreasing stress levels. Other researched benefits of meditation include reduced inflammation, improved immunity, and reduced risk of heart disease, stroke, and even cancer.

TRY MEDITATION

There is no "perfect" setting for meditating as long as you feel comfortable. If you don't already practice meditation, I'd like you to set a goal to do so, for just a few minutes each day. Here are some tips and ideas to get you started:

- **Focus on a single point:** Notice your breath, pick a single word or an affirmation, stare at a flame, listen to a gong or piece of music, or count beads on a mala (beaded necklace). Start doing this for a few minutes, and slowly increase the length of time you bring your awareness to a particular object.
- **Walk to meditate:** If sitting still doesn't feel meditative for you, the practice of walking meditation takes you out in nature to quietly observe your surroundings, so that your thoughts become part of the background, and you find yourself fully present in your environment.
- **Use a guide:** There are many podcasts and apps that offer guided meditations to help you meditate. A voice may guide you in visualizing specific mental imagery, or it may walk you through a series of breathing exercises and mantras to help you practice meditating. Popular apps include Headspace, Calm, and Insight Timer.
- **Learn from a master:** You may be interested in learning unique meditation techniques and approaches from well-respected leaders in the field. I've heard from many people who have decreased stress, lessened anxiety, and improved sleep with the Ziva Technique developed by Emily Fletcher.

- **Use a device:** The Muse brain-sensing device, which tracks your brain activity, heart rate, breathing, and body movements while meditating. When you wear this tool as a headband, you'll get real-time feedback on your brain activity, which will guide your meditation experience and keep you focused!

  My favorite way to meditate is to simply focus on my breath. I close my eyes, sit in a relaxing place, and breathe in, and then breathe out, for five to fifteen minutes.

Biofeedback

Through auditory and visual feedback, we can learn to recognize the physical signs of stress—rapid heart rate, muscle tension, perspiration—and control our reactions, like breathing more deeply, to quiet the stress response. HeartMath is a type of biofeedback that uses different patterns of heart activity to help us shift from a sympathetic state into a parasympathetic one.

Neurofeedback

What if we could train the brain to calm down, shifting more easily from stress mode into relaxation mode, and thus making us less vulnerable to the stress symptoms such as anxiety, depression, brain fog, and poor sleep? Research suggests that neurofeedback, also called EEG biofeedback or neurotherapy, can do just that. It works by monitoring brain waves and "rewarding" positive brain activity with pleasant audio and video while brain wave activity indicating rising stress results in negative feedback, such as lowering the volume on the music. The brain craves the rewarding, positive feedback and so over time learns to self-correct when it veers into a fight-or-flight response and stay in better balance. Neurofeedback uses the brain's incredible ability to adapt and change, called neuroplasticity, to teach the brain healthier patterns and responses. Benefits include better focus, reprocessing traumas, improved sleep, and less anxiety. I love the NeurOptimal system and have found it incredibly helpful for reprogramming my stress response.

Safety Signal #3: Create Healthy Coping Strategies for Your Triggers

When we allow people, situations, or trauma to trigger us, we give away our power, letting our past experiences control how we feel and react in the present and shaping our future. Being triggered keeps us in a rigid and inflexible state—but we don't have to stay that way. We can use our triggers as a springboard for a change and a way to build resilience. Every time we respond differently to a trigger, we rewire our brains for healthier patterns.

If you believe that you will find a discussion of emotional triggers traumatizing for you, please skip to page 226.

What's a Trigger Anyway?

More than being rubbed the wrong way, triggers are certain actions or situations that set off a memory of a past trauma or portion of a traumatic experience. Keep in mind that any distressing, disturbing, or painful event or experience can be the source of trauma, from illness and injury to growing up with highly critical parents. Triggers incite an intense emotional or physical reaction from us. You may feel like screaming, crying, or lashing out. Or, maybe you want to run away, withdraw, and hide your hurt feelings. No matter how you specifically react—sadness, anger, anxiety, panic, or another emotion—triggers stimulate an overwhelming, strong emotional reaction and distress. In some cases, a trigger causes a flashback, a vivid memory that takes us out of the present moment and makes us feel as if we are experiencing the trauma all over again.

Triggers come in many forms: words, sounds, smells, sights, a person, location, memory, emotion (vulnerability, loneliness), or physical sensation (pain, muscle tension). They can stem from childhood experiences, such as the emotional abuse, neglect, and household dysfunction of adverse childhood experiences (ACEs) (discussed on page 49), or more recent events. Remember, any overwhelming experience could be the source of trauma.

One of the most challenging aspects of managing triggers is that they can occur at any time or place in everyday life. Sometimes, they may be predictable, such as connected to a specific holiday, anniversary, or activity. In my case, I was in a traumatic car accident on my way home from college where my tire popped and I swerved into oncoming traffic on a busy three-lane highway. I miraculously survived with only a case of whiplash. However, I was triggered at the thought of driving on the highway again and would avoid highways whenever possible. One time my friend asked me to drive him somewhere, and I didn't realize we would need to get on a highway. My reaction was very extreme. I shut down and wasn't able to function. I was overcome with panic and a cold sweat and started crying uncontrollably. I had to pull over and have my friend drive my car instead. The reaction was obvious and had an understandable connection to my accident, but there isn't always such a clear link. Triggers can be surprises that occur seemingly out of the blue, and can present in a variety of ways, setting off our fight-or-flight response.

How to Cope with Triggers

Triggers can control and sabotage our lives if we don't find healthy ways to resolve them by letting go of the trauma attached to them or find positive ways to cope with the emotions that they raise in us.

Hopefully when you get to addressing triggers, you will already have created some space for healing and reflection to allow you to shift the automatic responses that come with triggers.

Letting go of past experiences may be simple, or it may require deep work involving psychotherapy or other counseling methods that may take a long time. (We'll cover ways to release trauma later in this chapter.) But we can take the following three steps to start coping with our triggers in a healthier way and build up our resilience.

Step One: Identify Your Triggers

Identifying our triggers is the first step in figuring out how best to cope with challenging situations. When you experience strong feelings of anxiety, panic, sadness, or anger, reflect on what is really happening. What may have led to those feelings? Was it something someone said, or a particular event that precipitated the rush of negative emotions? A pattern may emerge that suggests a potential trigger. Triggers are also as unique and individual as we are. What triggers one person may not trigger another. For one person, feeling unappreciated could be a trigger, while for another, feeling like someone is trying to control them may set them off. If your triggers are difficult to identify, working with a therapist may be helpful to identify your triggers.

Take a moment to identify your triggers. It may help to think back on the last few times when you felt frustrated, withdrawn, or ashamed; felt less than; got into a heated argument with another person; or lost your cool.

Describe a situation when you were triggered.

Example: My husband told me that I exceeded our budget on my shopping trip and I got mad and yelled at him to mind his business.

What feelings did the situation bring up for you?

Example: I felt like my husband was trying to control me and didn't appreciate my contribution to our household.

What are the triggers that became apparent from this situation?

Example: Feeling like someone is trying to control me, feeling underappreciated

Step Two: Recognize Your Coping Mechanisms

You may already have some coping mechanisms you lean on to help calm you down and shift your emotional state when you're triggered. Most of us do! In a triggered moment, when you're overwhelmed and want to blow your top or are consumed with anxiety, what do you do?

Some coping mechanisms are healthy and lead to positive results in the short and long term. They can lessen the impact of the trigger by making us aware of what is happening. Then we can diffuse the trigger's power over us

and regain control of our emotions. Positive coping mechanisms are beneficial because they return us to the present moment, reduce stress, and encourage a sense of calm. Triggers tend to thrust us back into a painful past.
But mindfulness practices such as taking deep breaths, journaling, practicing
meditation, and other grounding activities such as going for a hike, working
out, and petting your dog can help reconnect us with the here and now and
allow us to take deliberate control of our thoughts and emotions without
becoming overwhelmed by them. Healthy coping mechanisms give us a
chance to do the deeper work of processing our trauma when we're ready
and able.

Unhealthy (negative) coping mechanisms tend to numb us and distract
us from the present moment, masking the stress and difficult emotions in a
way that only makes the stress worse over time and creating new problems.
We often come to regret these coping mechanisms. Examples include:

- Aggressions or violent outbursts (hitting someone, throwing or kicking
  something, verbal abuse)
- Drinking alcohol, smoking, or doing drugs
- Overeating
- Overspending
- Self-harm
- Withdrawing from social contact (watching television, using social
  media, oversleeping, overworking)

In my college days, I smoked cigarettes to cope with my triggers. I even
won an award in my sorority for being "the pledge most likely to sit outside
and smoke cigarettes." When someone said or did something that made me
angry, I would go outside and smoke a cigarette. Deep down, I knew the
cigarettes didn't really make me feel better, and of course, I knew cigarettes
were bad for my body, but yet it was a coping mechanism.

After a certain point, reaching for a cigarette in an overwhelming moment was just an automatic reflex. During pharmacy school, I decided to
quit smoking for good. I felt like a big hypocrite as a smoker, advising people
on their health! I realized that I was reaching for a cigarette anytime I was
unable to process my feelings of being sad, angry, rejected, stressed, or

lonely. It wasn't until I became more consciously aware of my coping mechanisms that I was able to recognize how much mine were working against me.

One afternoon, after my fiancé (now my husband) and I had a fight and I stormed out of the house, I realized I had a choice between doing something that would worsen or improve my health. I could drive to the gas station and buy cigarettes and a lighter, or I could drive to the grocery store and pick out healthy foods and learn to cook a new meal. I chose the latter. Since that time I haven't smoked, and I have made tiny little steps like this at various crossroads to transform my life. Smoking was obviously working against me! Again and again. I was caught in a cycle of self-destructive behavior that harmed me physically, emotionally, and psychologically by preventing me from dealing with what triggered me in the first place.

Breaking the cycle meant first acknowledging the harmfulness of the behavior and then replacing it with a healthy coping mechanism. These days, I limit my triggers and pad my life with enough space for healing and self-care to allow for that pause. I have also expanded my repertoire of coping mechanisms for those moments when I do get triggered. I hope you can do the same.

I encourage you to consider your coping mechanisms now. What are the coping mechanisms you use to respond to the triggers you identified in Step One?

_____

_____

_____

_____

_____

_____

Do you think they are working for you or against you? How so?

_____

_____

_____

_____

_____

_____

Step Three: Change How You Respond to Triggers

There's no single way to self-soothe or get yourself back in balance after being triggered. But if you're using negative coping mechanisms, consider replacing them with more positive habits and routines.

- **Trigger:** Sally comes home after a long day at the office anxious about work tasks left undone and a long list of household chores to do. She wants to spend time with her children before they go to bed and worries she's not giving them enough attention. She's putting a load of laundry into the washing machine while helping her son with his math homework when her partner comes home and asks, "What's for dinner?" sending her stress level into the stratosphere.
- **Current coping mechanism:** Sally immediately pours herself a glass of wine to help calm her down and make it through the next few hours before bedtime. The wine makes her sleepy, but she wakes up around 2 a.m. and can't fall back to sleep, leaving her tired and irritable the next day.
- **Space for healing and new coping mechanisms:** On her commute home, Sally listens to soothing, relaxing music. At home in the evenings, when her stress begins to boil over, she takes a few deep, centering breaths, does a quick stretch, or brews a cup of tulsi tea to return to balance. Instead of checking work emails before bed, she spends fifteen minutes knitting a baby blanket she's making for her sister's newborn.

Sometimes we can avoid triggering situations, but that's not always possible—or helpful. The "before children" me would recommend getting a babysitter when a parent needed a break. Now, as a mom, I know that's not always realistic, or even the best thing to do at the moment.

That's why it's good to have a variety of positive coping mechanisms in your "trigger tool kit." You'll find that some practices work better in certain situations than others. It may help you to keep a list of the strategies you think will work well for you so that when you find yourself in need of relief, you have a ready resource to scan and can quickly choose the approach that seems most appealing to you at that time. Having a plan for the next time you get triggered will help you get through that situation with much more grace and ease, and much less heartache and pain.

What are some new coping mechanisms you could use to replace the ones that are no longer serving you?

_____

_____

_____

_____

_____

_____

_____

_____

_____

_____

_____

_____

_____

_____

_____

_____

_____

_____

_____

_____

Develop Your Trigger Tool Kit
Consider adding any of the oxytocin-boosting strategies from Chapter 6, as well as strategies mentioned in this chapter, such as moving your body or slowing your breath, to your trigger tool kit of de-stressing and mindfulness

techniques, which can shift you into a parasympathetic state when you are triggered:

- Inhale the fragrance of lavender essential oil.
- Hug a loved one (ideally one who is not the source of your trigger). ☺
- Pet your dog or cat.
- Take a bath.
- Get a massage.
- Journal your feelings.
- Create something new.
- Spend time in nature.
- Move your body.
- Meditate.
- Pray.
- Use affirmations.

My favorite affirmations and thoughts to ponder when triggered are:

- I feel angry, but I am not my anger.
- Never take criticism from someone you don't want to emulate.
- In the grand scheme of things, is this really important?
- What is the lesson I can learn from this?
- How do I want to show up in the world?
- What am I grateful for?
- Will I let this ruin my day?
- And the old Polish proverb, "Not my circus, not my monkeys."

Here are some additional practices I encourage you to try. (Special thanks to my friend Steve Wright of the Healthy Gut Project for giving me so much insight around this topic!)

- **Take deep breaths with auditory exhales:** Breathing in a deep, even rhythm while engaging your diaphragm, so that your belly rises and falls with each breath, turns off the fight-or-flight response and turns on the rest, relax, and recovery mode controlled by the parasympathetic nervous system. In addition to calming the physical body, this type of breathing quiets the mind by bringing focused attention to the breath. Exhale audibly to savor the most relaxing part of each breath and fully "let go." One of my favorite techniques is the 4-7-8 exercise, developed by Dr. Andrew Weil. With this breathing pattern, you breathe in through your nose for a count of 4, hold your breath for a count of 7, and then breathe out through your mouth for a count of 8.
- **Pause for a moment:** Be in the present moment and notice your surroundings. Try these techniques to help you:
  - Look around you. Identify one thing you can see, one thing you can touch, one thing you can hear, one thing you can smell, and one thing you can taste.
  - Get a breath mint (one that is free of inflammatory ingredients, of course) or ripe blueberry. Notice how it looks, feels, and smells. Put it in your mouth and roll it around, noticing the sensations.
  - Splash some water on your face. Notice how the water feels against your skin and the texture of the towel as you dry off. Use words in your mind to describe your impressions.
- **Talk with a trusted, supportive friend, family member, or therapist:** Tapping into your social support network to talk about your problems, validate your feelings, feel less alone, and gain useful advice or valuable perspectives can bring many benefits, including an effective buffer against the negative effects of stress. Aim to practice authentic sharing, openly and honestly communicating your inner reality to others while being open to gaining new insight and advice on how to manage the cause of what you're feeling going forward.
- **Move:** Dance and shake it off. Do some yoga. Go for a hike! Moving your body amps up the production of endorphins, chemicals produced by the nervous system that trigger a positive feeling by interacting with the receptors in your brain to reduce your perception of pain and

stress. Peter A. Levine, PhD, who developed somatic therapy (page 235), realized that animals in the wild who "freeze" under threat when fight-or-flight isn't an option release the massive amount of pent-up energy generated by the stress response by shaking and trembling. If that energy isn't released, the body considers itself still under threat.

- **Use visualization:** Instead of focusing on the panic, anxiety, anger, or sadness released by a trigger, close your eyes, and use your imagination to turn your attention to a calming, pleasurable image such as a white, sandy beach, large open field of flowers, a beautiful mountain lake, or another scene that relaxes you. Stay with that image until you've returned to balance, your mind and body are quiet, and you can return to the present moment refreshed. Guided visualizations are widely available to help walk you through the process—I encourage you to give them a try. In one study, women with fibromyalgia who practiced guided imagery on a daily basis for ten weeks reported a significant decrease in their feelings of stress, fatigue, pain, and depression compared to those who did not do it.

- **Shift your perspective:** When someone is challenging or judging me and I feel triggered, I have found it very healing to tap into my empathy and to play devil's advocate to see the world through their eyes. Empathy doesn't mean agreeing with the person's words or actions (not likely!) but rather allowing that they have a different point of view. It is an antidote to the anger, irritation, and resentment that can bubble up in these situations and works really well with my toddler son, parents, and other people whom I love, as well as people I'm not close to.

In my personal experience and my time working with clients, I have come to feel that identifying our triggers and coping mechanisms offers an opportunity for introspection, personal growth, and self-love. Taking some time to support ourselves in a positive, healing way after a triggering episode is one of the best ways we can become more resilient. These practices can help us as we approach some of the deeper work associated with addressing triggers and building resilience, such as forgiveness.

PUTTING IT ALL TOGETHER:
MY NEW COPING MECHANISMS

Use the prompts in this chart to help you review your current triggers and coping mechanisms and identify positive replacements. Write your own answers in your journal.

My Trigger	Current Coping Mechanism	Why It's No Longer Serving Me	New Replacement Coping Mechanism
I feel exhausted when x happens.	I reach for caffeine.	I can't sleep at night because I get too wired.	Drink a refreshing beverage like water mixed with electrolytes.
I feel frustration when y happens.	I reach for wine.	I feel hungover the next morning.	Drink a relaxing tea like tulsi.

I've seen firsthand that some of our adaptive thought patterns and behaviors that once helped us to survive but are no longer needed can prevent long-term adrenal balance—in my own journey and also with my clients. We're creatures of habit, and it's easy to fall back into the same old patterns again and again. This program is meant to help you change some of those ingrained thought and behavior patterns that helped you survive then but no longer serve you or weigh you down now.

For example, the same habits that got me through my doctoral program in pharmacy school that were necessary to keep up with all of my classes and exams (studying all day and night, wearing sweats every single day, hardly ever showering, and never leaving the house unless going to class or work) were not the same behaviors that helped me meet my soulmate (this was at a time when online dating was still in infancy, so yes, I actually had to leave my house to meet him). Shedding the patterns that no longer serve you and instilling new healing habits can transform your health and your life.

Just as we need to move out of our physical comfort zone to build muscle, we need to move out of our mental comfort zone to build mental resilience. So far I have shared so many ways to shift your body out of the stress

**When you know you need
to do some trauma work,
but instead you just use
positive affirmations...**

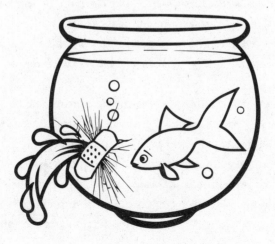

response into a healing parasympathetic state. Consider these strategies your foundation while you do some deeper healing work.

I love the proverb "Trust in God, but tie your camel." You don't have to be religious or even own a camel to appreciate this quote. The quote reminds me that just as we need to focus on our thoughts, we also need to take action. Just as it's important to use positive affirmations and positive self-talk, we also need to do some deeper healing work that will focus on addressing the underlying issues on why we are triggered in the first place. The saying goes: If you only trust in God, your camel might run away; if you only tie your camel, you will be anxious. If you only use positive affirmations, you may not get to the root cause of why you may be stuck in habits that aren't serving you, and if you only focus on the deep, heavy work, without the revitalizing safety signals, you may become overwhelmed.

Safety Signal #4: Let Go of the Heaviness That Weighs You Down

Many of us carry the heaviness of resentment, limiting beliefs, and trauma that keeps us stuck in a fight-or-flight state and prevents us from healing. When we let go of it, we not only release the stress and tension weighing us down, we make room in our lives for people and experiences that uplift and support us.

Forgive Everything and Everyone—Including Yourself

You may have heard that resentment is like drinking poison and hoping the other person will die. Carrying resentments around can feel like we're lugging around a five-pound bag of potatoes everywhere we go (thank you, HeatherAsh Amara, author of *Warrior Goddess Training*, for this perfect simile!).

In one study, participants who were asked to ruminate on someone who had hurt, mistreated, or offended them demonstrated significant signs of stress, including increased blood pressure and heart rate, facial tension, and sweating. When asked to practice forgiveness, their stress levels returned to those of normal wakefulness. In addition to triggering a heightened stress response, unforgiveness may compromise the immune system in many ways, including throwing off hormone production and the ability of cells to fight off infection. Beyond the physical impact, resentments may negatively influence other relationships and experiences, making it difficult to enjoy the present because we are dwelling on the past.

Forgiveness, the conscious decision to let go of the animosity, rage, and other emotions associated with the act that hurt you, lifts the burden of these negative emotions from our shoulders. Studies have linked forgiveness to a range of physical, mental, and emotional health benefits, including reduced anxiety, better sleep, and a greater sense of well-being and empowerment.

I struggled with forgiveness until I realized that forgiveness is for our own benefit, not for the benefit of the people who hurt us. Forgiveness frees us from the emotional "baggage" we've been carrying. It's important to note that forgiving someone does not mean we have to "make up" with them, allow them to hurt us again, or excuse the harm their actions have caused. That's why forgiveness doesn't require you to have contact with the person who injured you and is also possible even if the person who has hurt you has died or is no longer in your life.

In addition to carrying resentment for others, many of us carry guilt over something we did or didn't do. When it comes to reflecting on past actions, we must realize that most of us make the best decisions we can with the information we have at the time. In some cases, we get more information after the fact, or our eyes open to a truth that we were not aware of previously. Forgiving ourselves for our regrets over things we "should" have done can often be more difficult than forgiving others . . . but forgiving ourselves is just as important, and perhaps even more important than forgiving others.

Forgiveness is a process that often involves:

- Identifying the hurts you are carrying.
- Acknowledging your emotions about the hurt and harm done to you.
- Recognizing the ways carrying this burden has affected you.
- If you're ready, choosing to release those feelings and forgive.
- Marking this intention with an action, such as expressing your feelings in a safe way in a journal or by speaking with a trusted, supportive loved one, mentor, or therapist.

- Considering professional support. Some hurts, especially traumas, are more challenging to forgive than others and don't need to be faced alone.

FOR REFLECTION:
FORGIVING OURSELVES AND OTHERS

Consider using these exercises to expand your journaling practice:

1. I love the liberating act of writing out the things "I should have done," as well as things "I was not able to do then." This is a powerful reframe and step toward forgiving ourselves from David Hawkins, author of many books on self-empowerment, including *Letting Go*. Try it for yourself.

I should have . . .	I was not able to do then . . .
I should have been more supportive of my sister during her divorce.	*I was not able to be present for her then, but I can take steps to improve our relationship now.*

2. List all of the resentment, anger, hurt, and sadness that you carry around. What next steps can you take toward releasing them? (For help, refer to the process of forgiveness on page 227.)

_____

_____

_____

_____

_____

EMOTIONAL ABUSE

Too many of us tolerate emotional abuse, a consistent pattern of words and actions aimed at controlling and undermining another person through criticism, shame, manipulation, and embarrassment. We tend to think of abuse as physical and will often just take emotional abuse because our Western culture states: "Sticks and stones may break my bones, but words will never hurt me." I think this "be tough" mentality is contributing to our issues with mental health, burnout, and chronic illness. This is very black-and-white thinking . . . abuse is a spectrum.

Emotional abuse can wound in many ways, from feelings of self-doubt and worthlessness to high levels of inflammation in the body. Tensions and conflicts in a toxic relationship create a constant state of fight-or-flight, with studies showing strife, threat, isolation, and rejection leading to elevated markers of inflammation and that people in relationships with high levels of hostility exhibit the highest increases in inflammation. Removing inflammatory people from our lives is just as important as removing inflammatory foods! Keep in mind, emotional abuse can be directed at us from anyone: a significant other, family member, friend, or co-worker/boss.

While emotional abuse can sometimes be so subtle it can be hard to detect, always remember: You deserve to be treated with kindness and respect! Some signs of emotional abuse are:

- Lack of support
- Put-downs and name-calling
- Jealousy
- Controlling behaviors
- Dishonesty
- Ignoring your needs or wishes
- Isolation from friends and family
- Feeling drained after spending time together

Stop Tolerating

Do you feel like you put up with or tolerate a lot of behavior and situations in your life that actually annoy you? Many of us do. We keep quiet and don't do or say anything to address them and the frustration we feel builds up and up. For example, maybe you tolerate:

- Clutter on the floor
- Criticism from loved ones
- Lateness or disrespect for your time
- Passive-aggressive comments from a co-worker
- Pointless, never-ending meetings
- Lack of appreciation for your efforts

A huge transformation in my life occurred when I got rid of all of the things I was tolerating and started living my life on my terms. You may think, *Sure, the pile of dirty dishes in the sink annoys me but it's no big deal.* But once you start thinking about all of the "little" frustrations throughout your day, you'll find those little things add up to a lot. Many of us have dozens, hundreds, thousands (!) of these irritations, and over time, they stress us out and drag us down . . . sometimes, until we snap.

Simply writing out everything that you are tolerating will declutter your mind and improve your awareness of those energy drains. This is the first step to fixing them, even if you may not be willing or able to do anything about them right now. For the ones you do wish to focus on now, make a plan. Some may have simple, straightforward solutions. Tackle that low-hanging fruit first and see how good it makes you feel! Others may take longer to work out. That's okay. Try to take one action at a time that moves you closer to clearing it up. One by one, step by step, knock your list down and clear these stressors from your daily life.

Of course, we can't get rid of every single source of stress in our lives, even temporarily. We will experience frustration from time to time. For those situations that we cannot change (traffic immediately comes to mind!), use your trigger tool kit to help you feel more relaxed.

Use this chart to help you.

I have been tolerating . . .	I plan to address it by . . .
Example: I have been tolerating my partner's expectations that I will clean the house every weekend.	*I plan to address this by:* *1. Sharing how overwhelmed this makes me feel.* *2. Suggesting we divide up the chores.* *3. Offering to find a cleaning service.*

Replace Negative Self-Talk and Limiting Beliefs

You may have an inner critic who is just downright cruel. (I prefer the term "gremlin," as coined by Rick Carson, author of *Taming Your Gremlin: A Surprisingly Simple Method for Getting Out of Your Own Way*.) This gremlin is full of blame, shame, and harsh words: *You never do anything right. You're not smart enough to get that job. No one will ever love you.* We know that positive self-talk, self-compassion, and affirmations lessen the effects of stress and build resilience, helping us to get and stay motivated to make the changes necessary to achieve our health and life goals. While affirmations can help significantly, to fully vanquish the gremlin for good, we need to get at the root and address the limiting beliefs feeding it.

Limiting beliefs are beliefs that we have about ourselves, the world, or other people that hold us back from achieving our purpose in life. By believing these inaccurate perceptions, we limit our own potential and place roadblocks in our path that make reaching our goals, including our health goals, seem unattainable.

Often, these beliefs are formed when we are children and are highly influenced by what we're told by our parents, caregivers, teachers, relatives, friends, advertising, and the media. The childhood brain is often likened to a sponge because of how receptive it is to outside influences. According to the research of Bruce Lipton, a stem cell biologist and bestselling author of *The Biology of Belief*, children under age six primarily operate in a brain state below consciousness. While they take in vast amounts of information about their environment, they don't yet have the capacity to consciously evaluate whether what they're taking in is true or not. We unconsciously accept what the people around us tell us and we don't yet have the cognitive capacity to challenge those beliefs and make our own determinations.

The beliefs other people hold can damage our sense of self and prospects. For example, children who were always told they were not good at speaking may grow up believing this to be true. They may avoid jobs that involve speaking to a large group, restricting their opportunities. Instead of pursuing their dream of becoming a CEO, they settle for work that is not as public-facing because of their "speaking problem." When their friends tell them that they are a great person to engage in conversation with, they may not believe them and think they are "just saying that."

These beliefs may serve us well up to a point. If, as a child, you felt your parents were proud of you only if you got good grades, you may have had an exceptional school record but, on the downside, come to believe that only by being "perfect" could you gain love and approval from others. As an adult, the perfectionist mindset could be the source of many seemingly unrelated problems such as anxiety, insomnia, and workaholism.

Here are other examples of limiting beliefs:

- I am not good (smart, young, pretty, thin, healthy, etc.) enough.
- I am not likable.
- I am not good with money.
- I do not deserve to be loved.

- I'm not good at X (working with numbers, cooking, making friends, etc.).
- I will always be sick.
- I don't know how to be organized.

Now that we're adults, we can consciously change our thinking, clearing out harmful limiting beliefs and replacing them with more positive and empowering ones. Awareness is the first step in transforming a limiting belief, but a key component is challenging the limiting belief by imagining or explaining how it may not be true. Consider the following steps to transform your limiting beliefs:

1. **Identify a limiting belief:** Consider areas where you feel challenged consistently. If you're always struggling in relationships, for example, that may be a sign of a limiting belief at work.
2. **Understand why you have the belief:** Try to identify the origin, often a painful emotional experience.
3. **Show yourself some compassion:** Allow yourself to feel the emotions attached to the limiting belief with kindness and compassion.
4. **Acknowledge how the belief is holding you back:** Reflect on how the limiting belief is impacting your relationships, career, and health journey.
5. **Challenge the belief:** Is it accurate? Does it even make sense? By questioning your limiting belief, you'll recognize how untrue it is and weaken it.
6. **Replace the belief with a more positive one:** Transform the limiting belief of your inner critic into a belief offered by a compassionate best friend viewing the same circumstances. For me, it helps to imagine how a compassionate Chewbacca might reply to critical Gremlin (voice and all), but admittedly I am a little weird. ☺

Here are some examples of exchanging a harmful limiting belief with a more realistic, empowering one. I encourage you to consider a growth mindset, and the power of "yet," as you work to shed these beliefs.

Critical Gremlin	Compassionate Chewbacca
Example: I can't do anything right.	I'm a capable person and I am doing my best.
Example: I hate my body.	I'm developing a healthier relationship with my body.
Example: I am so disorganized.	I'm not organized yet, but I am working on it.

By identifying the beliefs that we have identified as "truths," we can begin to examine them, diffuse the power they have over us, and replace them with positive beliefs that will propel us toward our goals. I believe you can let go of these limiting beliefs and further your healing journey!

Doing the work of personal transformation and replacing outdated coping mechanisms, emotions, relationships, and limiting beliefs with ones that support us can raise difficult and uncomfortable emotions, but there is hope as well as many healing modalities that can help us release them.

Releasing Trauma

Sometimes, trauma is weighing on us. If you have experienced anything traumatic in the past, working through trauma, often with a professional therapist, is critical for healing. Here are some strategies I recommend looking into with a qualified practitioner:

Trauma-focused cognitive behavioral therapy

Cognitive behavioral therapy is a type of talk therapy that seeks to improve quality of life by challenging and replacing unhelpful negative thought patterns, beliefs, and behaviors related to a past trauma. Changing a person's thinking and assumptions can lead to better coping skills and healthier behaviors. Studies support it as an effective treatment option for a range of traumas, including sexual assault, traffic accidents, natural disasters, and war, among others.

Somatic therapy

Also known as somatic experiencing, this therapy combines talk therapy with mind-body exercises, such as breath work, meditation, and other physical techniques, to release the stress, tension, and other emotions remaining in the body (somatic) because of past trauma. Somatic therapy works to help release that stored energy and quiet the stress response through a variety of techniques to get at the root cause of trauma symptoms. Research has shown it to be an effective treatment for PTSD.

Brain retraining programs based in neuroplasticity

Limbic retraining programs, like the Dynamic Neural Retraining System and Gupta Program Brain Retraining, tap into the brain's ability to change and adapt. Various exercises and stimuli train the brain to discard old, harmful patterns and create new, healing ones. Most of my clients who have tried these programs have found them to be life changing.

Eye movement desensitization and reprocessing (EMDR) therapy

Based on the observations and research of Francine Shapiro, PhD, an American psychologist and educator, EMDR is intended to change the way a traumatic memory is stored in the brain in order to lessen the vividness and emotion surrounding it, reducing stress. This is accomplished through a series of eye movements, directed by a therapist, while thinking about the painful memory. The EMDR method has been found to be equivalent in efficacy to trauma-focused cognitive behavior therapy and to be an evidence-based treatment for PTSD with lasting benefits, but in contrast to trauma-focused talk therapy that can take years, EMDR works quickly, and you may be able to see results in one to three sessions.

EMDR has helped me process several past traumas, including the terrible car accident I mentioned earlier and the sudden death of a loved one.

After a single one-hour session of EMDR, I was able to reprocess the car accident completely, and can now navigate even the busiest interstate stress-free. In contrast, the loss of a loved one took two full days of intensive therapy known as induced after-death communication (IADC), in which a variation of EMDR is used to help clients reconnect with their deceased loved ones and process their grief (in addition to a year of grief therapy). There are many different types of therapies available—this is by no means an exhaustive list. Consider one that appeals to you and best suits your needs.

Safety Signal #5: Reclaim Your Space by Setting Healthy Boundaries

For some people, the word "boundary" has a negative connotation, suggesting a wall separating ourselves from the people around us. Rather, boundaries are ways of strengthening our relationships by providing healthy rules for handling them. When we set boundaries, we are protecting ourselves and limiting our exposure to stress while being respectful to others and letting them know what they can expect from us. Perhaps most important, we are acknowledging our worth and that we are entitled to our own thoughts, feelings, opinions, personal space, friends, social activities, spiritual beliefs, and possessions (including money). A lack of boundaries, particularly between work and home life, takes a physical and emotional toll. Added stress is just one result. Studies have linked blurred boundaries to emotional exhaustion, unhealthy lifestyle behaviors, reduced happiness, and a greater risk of family conflict.

Setting Healthy Boundaries

Where do you end and where do I begin? Being able to set and enforce boundaries, what you will and will not put up with, is one of the most useful skills to have once we decide to let go of what's weighing us down. Often, by establishing or reinforcing a boundary around our time, personal space, and belongings, we can remove some of those daily irritations contributing to an overworked stress response. In fact, irritation and resentment frequently signal that some boundary building would be beneficial. Other signs include:

- Drama! Where there's frequent upheaval and conflict, there is a need for boundaries.
- Feeling depleted, anxious, or wound up.
- Being swamped with inconvenient obligations and overburdened by the demands of others.

The boundaries we currently hold have been shaped by many aspects in our life—starting from birth. In other words, our boundaries develop based on the family dynamics we grew up with, where we live, our culture and heritage, and whether we identify as an introvert, extrovert, or even a bit of both. But, even though our boundary standards are shaped throughout our childhood, we do not have to stick to those specific boundaries. We can change them at any time to better suit our current needs. For example, you may have felt comfortable answering questions from your work colleagues about your upcoming wedding, but you do not want to discuss your health with them. It's natural for your boundaries to evolve over time.

For some of us, setting boundaries comes naturally, while for others it's a struggle. The good news is, it is a skill all of us can develop and perfect with practice. Here are some ways to practice setting boundaries:

Say no

Did you know that "no" is a complete sentence? Say it with me: "No." Simple, short, and very effective. At the beginning of my healing journey with Hashimoto's, learning to set firm boundaries and especially to say no helped me stop stressing myself out at work. Instead of working nonstop, I took advantage of lunches, breaks, days off, flex time, working from home, and the company's policy that allowed scheduled sick days. I left the office on time. When I became overwhelmed with projects and people asked me to take on more, I said that magical word, "no"—and it felt good. For the first time in my adult life, I felt like I was in that mystical zone of "work-life balance." It's your right to say no; embrace it.

Be assertive

Express your boundary requests in a polite but firm manner. When we are assertive, we are not blaming or threatening another person but we are clearly stating what we want, with no room for negotiation. How can you be assertive without coming across as aggressive and inadvertently harm your relationship? Avoid blame and use statements that refer to you and your feelings.

For example:

- Aggressive: You need to start cleaning up your mess and help me with the house. You are so lazy!
- Assertive: I feel extremely overwhelmed when I have to spend an entire weekend cleaning the whole house by myself. I need time to rest and relax so I'm ready to start the week fresh. Can you help me by cleaning X, Y, and/or Z this weekend?

Protect your time

Do you often find that you are 100 percent available, every second of the day? Thanks to today's "convenient access" to our phones and other devices, most of us are always available by a quick text or email, resulting in us having little to no personal time. You can create boundaries for your time—and again, with no explanation—by:

- Scheduling your alone time. Put it on your calendar, and ensure you are in a place where you will not be disturbed by phones, computers, and visitors.
- Deleting any social media and email apps from your phone, or silencing their notifications.
- Using the "Do Not Disturb" mode on your phone. (Note: This mode allows you to identify contacts who can "disturb" you so you will not be out of reach to those who may need you, such as elderly parents and children.)
- Making a pact with yourself that you will not respond to emails, texts, etc., after a certain time of the day.
- Using "out of office" responders if you use email for work purposes.

Some people in your life may be shocked when you start setting or changing boundaries. Communication is key to prevent resentments from building. Be clear, firm, and respectful. Trust me, the more you practice setting boundaries, the better you'll get at it.

If you are having trouble setting boundaries or someone is making it difficult for you to set boundaries, perhaps because mental illness may be a factor, I encourage you to reach out to professionals for assistance. They can help you strategize the most effective ways to keep your boundaries respected.

Setting boundaries takes effort but it can be life changing! It is an important form of self-care, clearing out the drama, anger, and frustrations that build up when our limits are pushed and giving us the space to heal and grow.

FOR REFLECTION: SETTING BOUNDARIES

Consider using these prompts to expand your journaling practice:

I experience drama in these places in my life . . .

_____

_____

_____

_____

_____

_____

_____

I plan to start setting some boundaries by . . .

_____

_____

_____

_____

_____

_____

_____

I will create more personal time for myself by setting these boundaries . . .

_____

_____

_____

_____

_____

Action Steps

To rebuild resilience, aim to:

- Find ways to move your body that make you feel calm and relaxed (not exhausted).
- Try slowing your breath to shift from fight-or-flight mode into a healing, relaxed state.
- Replace unhealthy coping mechanisms with healthier ones that allow you space for healing.
- Let go of what no longer serves you by practicing forgiveness, ceasing to tolerate energy-sapping situations, replacing limiting beliefs, and releasing trauma. Feel your emotional load lighten!
- Give yourself the space to grow and heal by protecting your time with some healthy boundaries.

To view the scientific references cited in this chapter, please visit us online at https://thyroidpharmacist.com/atpbooknotes.

CHAPTER **8**

Review

Goal

• To complete the ATP with calm and confidence.

Sending your body safety signals over the next few weeks does not have to be overwhelming or complicated. Use the sample weekly schedules in If We Fail to Plan, We Plan to Fail in Chapter 3 (page 85) and the tools and quick reference guides in this chapter to make implementing every element of the program easy.

What's on the Menu?

Use this chart as a quick reference of which foods to remove and include during the program. Remember, the recipes included at the end of this book stay within these guidelines and offer simple, easy-to-prepare options for every meal and snack. You can use them as is or tweak them to better accommodate your preferences (while staying within the program guidelines).

Excluded Foods	Included Foods
Gluten Grains	All meats
Dairy (from all animals)	Low-glycemic vegetables
Soy	Low-glycemic fruit
High-glycemic vegetables	Eggs
High-glycemic fruit	Nuts (except peanuts, a legume)

Excluded Foods	Included Foods
Legumes (except green beans and pea protein)	Seeds
Refined sugar	Starchy vegetables (except white potato)
Seaweed	Black pepper (*Piper nigrum*)
Capsaicin-containing spicy peppers	Bell peppers
Alcohol	Healthy fats
Vegetable, canola, corn, soybean, cottonseed oils	Program-compliant protein powders
	Stevia, maple syrup, monk fruit, honey (in limited amounts)

Here's how an average day might look on the ATP diet.

The Adrenal Kick Start (page 297): It tastes like an orange Creamsicle, but has the benefits of boosting your morning glucose and vitamin C levels with organic orange juice (low glucose), lifting cortisol with sea salt, and setting you up for a stable blood sugar day with protein powder and high-fat coconut milk. You will drink it first thing in the morning (or thirty to sixty minutes after your thyroid medications if you take them).

Satisfying, simple-to-digest smoothies: Even if you're not typically hungry in the mornings, you will find that it's easy to shift your caloric intake to earlier in the day with tasty, nutrient-dense, and easy-to-digest smoothie options like the Root Cause Green Smoothie (page 304), Blueberry Pie Smoothie (page 303), or Adrenal Tonic Smoothie (page 303), or create your own, making sure to include these three components:

- **Fiber:** Include a variety of low-glycemic veggies, including leafy greens, and a small serving of berries for antioxidants.
- **Fat:** Coconut milk (full-fat) and avocado are great choices.
- **Protein:** Add one serving of a program-compliant protein powder to support blood sugar balance and get your daily recommended intake.

Nourishing, blood sugar–balanced lunches (salad/soup): We will keep
it simple with a big salad or soup made with plenty of healthy fats,
fiber, and protein. To keep the stress down, I love using the Mason Jar
Salad Hack below to prep and store my salads for the week.
(For a meal prep guide, go to thyroidpharmacist.com/atpbookbonus.)

- **Fat:** Use extra-virgin olive oil, olives, avocados, nuts, seeds, and
  coconut shavings.
- **Fiber:** Choose from the rainbow of low-glycemic veggies, such as
  bell peppers, cucumbers, broccoli, leafy greens, mushrooms, red
  onion, and tomatoes.
- **Protein:** Use cooked chicken or salmon, boiled egg, nuts, and seeds.

MASON JAR SALAD HACK

Set out five 32-ounce wide-mouth Mason jars, one for each weekday,
and get ready to stack the fruits and vegetables you've prepped!

- **Layer 1 (the bottom of the jar):** Everyday Dressing (page 305) or
  other ATP-compliant dressing of choice
- **Layer 2:** Firm vegetables, such as cut cucumber, bell peppers, or
  baby carrots
- **Layer 3:** Softer vegetables and fruit, such as olives, cherry
  tomatoes, or blueberries
- **Layer 4 (top layer):** Nuts or seeds, some greens, and coconut
  shavings or fresh herbs

  Seal and refrigerate. In the morning, grab a jar along with some
  protein or fat (chopped chicken or boiled eggs are some ideas for
  protein; avocados are great for fat) and take it with you for your
  lunchtime meal.

Easy, comforting, and easy to digest so you can rest dinners: Pair meats
and veggies for a satisfying dinner. You'll want the same balance of
healthy fats, fiber, and protein as with lunch. If you haven't gotten your
cruciferous vegetable in yet for the day, have them now. Cauliflower Mash

(page 327) is a favorite go-to side with dinner! To save time, many of my recipes feature the slow cooker and can be made in a pressure cooker.

In-between meals: In the early stages, as you work on stabilizing your blood sugar and circadian rhythm, you may benefit from strategic uses of fat- and protein-filled snacks, including caffeine-free, high-fat adaptogenic lattes; nutrient-dense, blood sugar–balancing juices mixed with fats; and/or caffeine-free healing teas.

- Fat- and protein-filled snacks (see Snacks, below)
- Mid-morning and midday slump-busting adaptogenic caffeine-free lattes (Maca Latte [page 300] and Tulsi Tea Latte [page 302])
- Nutrient dense, blood sugar–stabilizing juices mixed with fats (Adrenal Kick Start [page 297])
- A choice of caffeine-free teas tailored to your needs (Balancing Teas [page 161])

SNACKS

It's a good idea to keep low-carbohydrate snacks on hand to balance blood sugar and beat cravings. Check out the snacks included in the Recipes section, or mix and match from this list of my favorite blood sugar–stabilizing sources of fats and proteins to make your own delicious snacks:

Avocados	Nuts (except peanuts)
Chia seeds	Olives and extra-virgin olive oil
Chicken	Pea protein
Coconut	Pork
Coconut milk	Salmon
Duck fat	Sardines
Eggs and egg white proteins	Seeds
(if not sensitive)	Tallow
Grass-fed beef	Turkey
Hydrolyzed beef protein	Whitefish
Lamb	

Modifications for Your Unique Cortisol Curve

In Chapter 3 (page 83), I shared how to tune in to your symptoms to identify if you have low cortisol and need to emphasize cortisol-boosting activities, high cortisol and need to prioritize cortisol-lowering activities (and skip cortisol boosters), or fall somewhere in the middle and are on a cortisol roller coaster. Use your findings to determine which of the following refinements to the program will best support your healing.

Low Cortisol	Cortisol Roller Coaster	High Cortisol
Add the adaptogen licorice (recommended as part of an adrenal support supplement), grapefruit, and more salt to your diet to stretch out cortisol and support blood pressure in the morning and early afternoon.	Consider using these therapies if you have morning/afternoon fatigue, but avoid if you have high blood pressure.	Avoid licorice (recommended as part of an adrenal support supplement), grapefruit, and adding more salt to your diet, as they can increase your cortisol levels and blood pressure further.
Prioritize using bright lights in the morning and afternoon to boost cortisol naturally.	You will likely need to prioritize both using bright lights in the morning and afternoon and blocking bright lights and blue lights after sunset to help with normalizing your cortisol production.	Prioritize blocking bright lights and blue lights after sunset to prevent additional increased cortisol from bright light.
Avoid aerobic exercise, as it can make those with low cortisol feel tired and further reduce cortisol levels.	You may be able to tolerate aerobic exercise, but you may need to find an optimal time to exercise, as aerobic exercise may promote relaxation and balance or make you more tired, depending on the cortisol levels at the time of day you do it.	Aerobic exercise may promote relaxation and balance.

A Sample Day on the Adrenal Transformation Protocol

Use this sample schedule to help you optimally time the replenishing and reenergizing safety signals.

Food, Supplement, Hydration, and Circadian Safety Signals

Time	Safety Signals
7 a.m. (or your usual wake-up time)	· Adrenal Kick Start (page 297) · Begin the day out in the sunlight for at least thirty minutes. Go for a brisk walk, sip tea while journaling, or simply relax outside. · If you can't get outside, sit under a lamp that mimics sunlight for thirty minutes. · If you take thyroid medications first thing in the morning, wait 30 minutes before having anything to eat, drink, and/or taking supplements.
8 a.m., Breakfast	· Smoothie with protein powder (see pages 303–304 for suggestions) · Adrenal Support supplement · Carnitine, morning dose · Electrolytes · *Saccharomyces boulardii,* morning dose
10 a.m., Snack	· Latte/Green Juice/Snack/Herbal Tea (see pages 299–303 and 330–333 for suggestions)
12 p.m., Lunch	· Soup/Salad (see pages 305–310 for suggestions) · Eat in a light/bright place, preferably outside. · Take a walk now or later in the afternoon. Get as much sunlight throughout the day as possible!
3 p.m., Snack	· Latte/Green Juice/Snack/Herbal Tea (see pages 299–303 and 330–333 for suggestions)
6 p.m., Dinner	· Dinner (see pages 311–324 for suggestions) · Myo-inositol · Carnitine, evening dose · *Saccharomyces boulardii,* evening dose
7 p.m., Winding down	· Avoid electronic devices (TV, phone, computer) for one to two hours (the more the better!) before bedtime. · If you need to use a device, consider putting it in "nighttime" mode or wear blue light–blocking glasses, such as TrueDark eyewear. · Dim the lights in your house. Some people even use candles!
8 p.m., Snack	· Relaxing Tea (or Snack if needed)
9 p.m., Bedtime	· Magnesium supplement · Turn off all night lights. · Use blackout curtains or blinds to block light from outside. Put black tape over appliances with lights, such as humidifiers, chargers, and smoke detectors. I like TrueDark Junk Light Dots. · Sleep

Supplement Summary

These six supplements plus protein powder are my go-to recommendations for restoring adrenal balance and accelerating healing. Targeting the most common imbalances present with adrenal issues, these supplements contain the top adrenal-supporting nutrients and offer multiple healing benefits.

Supplement	Description	How to Use	Preferred Products	Notes for Nursing Moms
Adrenal Support Blend	A mixture of adaptogenic herbs, vitamins, and the amino acid tyrosine to support the adrenals. Blends that contain ashwagandha should be avoided by people with nightshade sensitivity. Blends with licorice should be avoided by those who have high blood pressure and/or high cortisol.	Once daily at breakfast. Start with one capsule and work your way up to three. Take thirty minutes to one hour after thyroid medication.	Rootcology Adrenal Support (contains licorice), Designs for Health Adrenotone (contains licorice), Pure Encapsulations Daily Stress Formula (licorice-free) (All of the brands listed contain ashwagandha.)	Not recommended. Consider stand-alone adaptogens, holy basil, shatavari, reishi, rhodiola, and +/- Pure Encapsulations B-Complex Plus (see Tired Mommy Protocol on page 272 for dosing).
Magnesium	Balances the adrenals, reduces pain, and promotes restful sleep. The citrate salt helps promote bowel movements. Reduce dose or switch to magnesium glycinate if diarrhea occurs.	1 teaspoon or two capsules daily at bedtime. Take four hours after thyroid medication.	Rootcology Magnesium Citrate Powder, Designs for Health MagCitrate Powder, Pure Encapsulations Magnesium (citrate/malate) Capsules, or Pure Encapsulations Magnesium Glycinate	Likely safe, but please check with your doctor/midwife before using.

Supplement	Description	How to Use	Preferred Products	Notes for Nursing Moms
Saccharomyces boulardii	Helps reduce gut inflammation and boosts our gut's own defense system. Can help reduce brain fog, blood sugar swings, anxiety, and joint pain. Should be avoided by those who have Crohn's disease.	One capsule, two times daily, at breakfast and dinner. Take thirty minutes to one hour after thyroid medication.	Rootcology *Saccharomyces boulardii*, Designs for Health Floramyces, Pure Encapsulations *Saccharomyces boulardii*	Likely safe, but please check with your doctor/midwife before using.
Myo-Inositol	Helps with blood sugar swings and can promote relaxation, as well as help those with OCD and PCOS. Should be used with caution in those with hypoglycemia, as it can reduce blood sugar.	¼ teaspoon, once per day, after dinner. Take thirty minutes to one hour after thyroid medication.	Rootcology Myo-Inositol Powder, Designs for Health Inositol Powder, Pure Encapsulations Inositol (powder)	Likely safe, but please check with your doctor/midwife before using.
Electrolytes	Helps balance electrolytes and keeps us hydrated. Contains high-dose vitamin C to support the immune system and nourish the adrenals and D-ribose to support energy levels.	1 scoop, once daily, at breakfast. (I like to add it to my smoothie.) Take four hours after thyroid medication.	Rootcology Electrolyte Blend, Designs for Health Electrolyte Synergy, Pure Encapsulations Electrolyte Energy Blend + Pure Encapsulations D-Ribose	Likely safe, but please check with your doctor/midwife before using.

Supplement	Description	How to Use	Preferred Products	Notes for Nursing Moms
Carnitine	Can help reduce thyroid-related fatigue. Can help balance blood sugar, convert fat inside our cells into energy, and reduce ammonia in the body (which can lead to brain fog). Look for blends that contain both L-carnitine and acetyl-L-carnitine, such as the Rootcology and Designs for Health recommended products.	Two capsules, twice daily, at breakfast and dinner.	Rootcology Carnitine Blend, Designs for Health Carnitine Synergy, Pure Encapsulations L-Carnitine	Likely safe, but please check with your doctor/midwife before using.

Protein Powders

You may benefit from adding protein powders to help ensure adequate protein intake.

Preferred Protein Brands

- Rootcology AIPaleo Protein
- Rootcology Paleo Protein (Vanilla)
- Rootcology Organic Pea Protein (Vanilla)
- Designs for Health PurePaleo Unflavored
- Designs for Health PurePaleo Vanilla
- Designs for Health Organic PurePea
- NOW Organic Pea Protein
- Manitoba Harvest Hemp Yeah! Max Protein Unsweetened Hemp Protein Powder

Protein powders are generally considered safe for nursing moms, but please check with your doctor or midwife.

Revitalizing Safety Signals

Each day, try to add one revitalizing activity (or more!) to your daily routine below. Start to incorporate resilience-building activities below around weeks 3 and 4.

Revitalizing Activities

- ☐ Journal.
- ☐ Use affirmations.
- ☐ Do an activity that makes you feel good.
- ☐ Hug—yourself or a loved one.
- ☐ Cuddle a pet, stuffed animal, or blanket.
- ☐ Get a massage.
- ☐ Do whatever makes you laugh.
- ☐ Inhale the fragrance of stress-relieving essential oils.
- ☐ Listen to uplifting music.
- ☐ Relax in a sauna.
- ☐ Take a warm bath with Epsom salt.
- ☐ Spend time in nature.
- ☐ Draw, paint, color, sew, bake—create!
- ☐ Exercise in a way that makes you feel good.
- ☐ Pray.
- ☐ Say yoga mantras, aloud or silently.
- ☐ Meditate.

Resilience-Building Safety Signals

Building resilience is deeper healing work that may take longer than the program and that's okay. The goal over these four weeks is to move forward in these areas, in whatever way feels good to you. I suggest adding resilience-building healing work after you've been doing daily revitalizing activities for at least one week.

Resilience-Building Healing Work

Step One: Pick one question from the following list:

☐ Do my coping strategies serve me?

☐ Am I carrying a hurt that could be forgiven?

☐ Am I tolerating behaviors or situations that frustrate me?

☐ Do I have a critical inner gremlin that shames and blames me with limiting beliefs?

☐ Do I need to set some healthy boundaries?

☐ Is trauma weighing me down?

Step Two: Decide to reflect, make a plan, or take action on that topic today.

☐ Reflect: Use your journal and the exercises and "For Reflection" prompts in the book to reflect on your thoughts and feelings.

☐ Make a plan: Determine the steps you could take to transform the situation.

☐ Take action: Move forward on one of the action steps you identified.

The Adrenal Transformation Protocol Checklist

This checklist will help you keep track of all you have accomplished on the program—and make sure you haven't inadvertently skipped anything!

On the ATP I've been . . .

Replenishing by:

☐ Following the ATP diet

☐ Supporting with the six core ATP supplements:

    ☐ Adrenal support

    ☐ Magnesium citrate

    ☐ *Saccharomyces boulardii*

    ☐ Myo-inositol

    ☐ Electrolyte blend

    ☐ Carnitine

Reenergizing by:

    ☐ Prioritizing proper hydration and electrolyte balance

    ☐ Supporting my mitochondria

    ☐ Resetting my circadian rhythm

Revitalizing by:

- ☐ Empowering myself with positive thought patterns
- ☐ Adding more pleasurable activities
- ☐ Boosting oxytocin
- ☐ Doing something creative

Rebuilding resilience by:

- ☐ Reclaiming my space by setting healthy boundaries
- ☐ Exercising in ways that support my healing
- ☐ Slowing my breath to calm the stress response
- ☐ Using healthy coping strategies when I'm triggered
- ☐ Letting go of the heaviness that weighs me down
- ☐ Practicing forgiveness
- ☐ No longer tolerating behavior and situations that annoy me
- ☐ Replacing negative self-talk and limiting beliefs
- ☐ Releasing trauma

Action Steps

- Don't sweat it! Refer to this chapter as you make your way through the four-week program to ease your way and keep you on track.

PART III

Next Steps and Advanced Protocols

CHAPTER **9**

Reassess and Move Forward

Hopefully, after completing the four-week ATP your symptoms have reduced significantly—or are even completely gone!—and you are feeling more like yourself again. I hope you're feeling energetic, strong, confident, calm, and like the real you has finally returned (or arrived)! It is my sincere hope that everything you've learned about sending your body safety signals to support a balanced stress response and build resilience has helped transform your health. In my experience, I've found that about 80 percent of participants feel 80 percent better in just these four weeks.

ATP SUCCESS STORIES

"The program has really changed how I feel energy wise. I'm not tired. I feel mentally clearer. I seem to have more resilience to stress and I feel a lot calmer. I've had more visions for the future and generally feel more excited about life."—CLAUDIA G.

"Most/Many of my symptoms are resolved. I finally gave myself permission to really rest. It has been years since I did any resting. . . . [A few] weeks is all you need to begin a healing journey. Hope becomes a certainty. I thought I would have to live with all the awful symptoms for the rest of my life, but I now can see a light at the end of a very long, dark tunnel!"—GERALDINE P.

"The ATP has changed my life. I was proud of myself because I was functioning on five to six hours of sleep each night. Actually, I found that not getting the proper amount of sleep each night was causing me adrenal imbalance. I no longer have brain fog, fall asleep midday, lack energy, or have acid reflux. I changed my sleep pattern and diet with the help of this program and the supplements were a big help in dealing with issues I was having with insulin intolerance and dehydration. I highly recommend this program. It changed my life."—DESIREE T.

Ideally, my goal is for 100 percent of people to see 100 percent reduction in each symptom, and for many of you, the fundamental protocols in the ATP will help you feel 100 percent better and ready to face each day with energy and enthusiasm, given enough time.

For others, these may be the first steps on your path to health and healing. If you're not improving a lot or have a few specific areas in need of more healing, don't give up! There is more we can do to get you closer to wellness.

How Are You Feeling Now?

Let's check in with how you're doing *now* so we can figure out your best next step. Have all of your symptoms improved or vanished? Do some symptoms still need work? After you've been able to implement the program for four weeks, review the Adrenal Assessment (page 69) you've (hopefully!) been filling out each week to track your symptoms over time and assess the current health of your adrenals. Hopefully, your total number of symptoms has significantly decreased or even resolved completely! Any remaining symptoms will help show you the way forward to feeling better.

- If all of your symptoms have resolved, you may most benefit from a maintenance plan, outlined in this chapter.
- If you are still experiencing adrenal imbalance symptoms, such as anxiety, brain fog, depression, fatigue, insomnia and sleep issues, low libido, and pain, you may most benefit from professional healthcare support, advanced testing, and the symptom-specific protocols outlined in Chapter 10.
- If most of your adrenal imbalance symptoms have resolved but you still don't feel like yourself, you may benefit from a deeper investigation

into your unique root causes and advanced testing and professional healthcare support. Use the Use Your Symptoms to Determine Your Next Step chart on page 261 to help you find the best resource for more root cause–digging and symptom solutions.

Please know that there is hope no matter which next step is best for you! Healing is a journey, not a race, and there is still so much more we can do to get a handle on all of your symptoms.

FUNDAMENTAL HEALING:
THE LIVER, ADRENALS, AND GUT

The body breaks down in predictable ways under stress. When we are stressed, our adrenals aren't the only part of the body to be affected. Chronic stress puts us more at risk for gut dysfunction, including a leaky intestinal barrier (leaky gut) and an imbalanced microbiome (gut dysbiosis), which compromise the gut's ability to detox and remove harmful waste from the colon.

That can strain the liver, the body's main detoxifier, and can call for extra support to improve its functionality. Sometimes, lingering symptoms after adrenal support can clue us in to whether the liver or gut is in need of more attention, but if you've been stressed for too long, you may need to address both in a comprehensive ninety-day plan.

You've already completed the four-week ATP, and in my book *Hashimoto's Protocol*, I share the two remaining pieces of the complete plan: my two-week Liver Support Protocol and six-week Gut Balance Protocol. Like the ATP, these protocols are broad-spectrum, meaning the self-directed lifestyle changes and targeted supplementation address multiple root causes and imbalances so you can start seeing profound improvements in multiple symptoms right away. Depending on your symptoms, these two protocols may be the support you need to feel significantly better.

Maintenance: If You Have Met Your Adrenal Health Goals

Whether you want to keep feeling as great as you do now or want to give the ATP a little while longer to clear more of your symptoms, you will benefit from incorporating these strategies into your day-to-day long term.

Many people report feeling better right away on the program, but even more report more energy, optimism, and health by carrying on with the program for more than four weeks. Habits take a while to really get cemented and sometimes, depending on the intensity of the symptoms, the body needs more time to reset. Consistency is often key to healing, and following the program long term might be a better way to reach your health goals.

Nourish

If you're feeling good on the diet, you may want to consider sticking with it until all of your symptoms are gone and then start to gradually reintroduce the foods you've eliminated. Follow my guidelines (How to Reintroduce Foods You've Eliminated, page 259) to make sure you identify your food sensitivities and don't reintroduce inflammatory foods.

If you have found the six ATP supplements and protein powder helpful, you may want to continue them for longer. (Refer to the chart on page 259 for the recommended duration of usage.) You may also decide to transition off these supplements.

Reenergize

The energy boost from supporting proper electrolyte balance and hydration, supporting the mitochondria, and living in sync with the circadian rhythm sells itself! Continue these diet and lifestyle strategies to extend the benefits. (See the chart on page 259 for the recommended duration of usage for the electrolyte and carnitine supplements.)

Revitalize

I hope that once you have seen just how powerful and transformative positive thought patterns, pleasurable activities, and creating are, these revitalizing strategies will become an essential part of your daily habits. Try to keep them as part of your routine and add in any additional ones that resonate with you.

Rebuild Resilience

Making sure we're treating ourselves with kindness and compassion while building resilience is an ongoing effort. Doing the deeper work of personal transformation can take time. Use what you've learned over the past few weeks to help you pay attention to more ways to be good to yourself and release inflammatory thoughts, people, and behaviors.

Use the Adrenal Transformation Protocol Checklist (page 251) to help make sure you're on track!

HOW LONG YOU CAN TAKE THE RECOMMENDED ADRENAL TRANSFORMATION SUPPLEMENTS

Adrenal Support Blend: Three months to two years, or as needed in times of increased stress

Carnitine: Three months or long term, as needed

Electrolytes with D-ribose: Long term

Magnesium: Long term

Myo-inositol: Six months or long term, as needed

Protein powders: Long term

Saccharomyces boulardii: Three months to two years

How to Reintroduce Foods You've Eliminated

The Adrenal Transformation diet is based on a Paleo diet that removes the most common food sensitivities seen in those with an impaired stress response and Hashimoto's. This diet should be followed until all of your symptoms have resolved. Then you can begin reintroducing foods into your diet.

The best way to return foods to your diet is gradually, starting with foods that are the least reactive. We'll reintroduce foods to your diet one by one and track your symptoms with each new addition for signs of a reaction. Make sure to only introduce whole foods so that you can pinpoint any reactions to that specific food. For example, if pizza is reintroduced, you will be reintroducing grains and dairy at the same time, along with any other toppings such as deli meats. Instead, it's best to introduce only one of those components, following the reintroduction list below. Please note, at this time, that there are three foods that usually continue to be problematic for most people, even with the use of my current protocols. Thus, I do not recommend that most people reintroduce soy, dairy, or gluten.

Food sensitivities can often manifest as any of the following symptoms:

Common Food Reactions

Body System	Symptoms
Lungs	Postnasal drip, congestion, cough, asthma
Gut	Constipation, diarrhea, cramping, bloating, nausea, gas, acid reflux, burning, burping
Heart	Increased pulse, palpitations
Skin	Acne, eczema, itchiness
Muscles	Joint aches, pain, swelling, tingling, numbness
Brain	Headaches, dizziness, brain fog, anxiety, depression, fatigue, insomnia

Step One

Reintroduce one eliminated food in limited amounts. Follow this order to proceed from the least to the most reactive foods:

1. Fruits
2. White potatoes
3. Grains (buckwheat, oats, quinoa, rice)
4. Legumes (e.g., chickpeas, kidney beans, black beans, pinto beans, peanuts, etc.)
5. Hot peppers/spices
6. Corn
7. Alcohol (spirits, wine, cider, gluten-free beer)
8. Deli meats
9. Ghee (if reintroducing dairy)
10. High-sugar sweeteners
11. Refined oils
12. Soy (soybeans, additives containing soy)

13. Dairy (if reintroducing)

14. Gluten-containing grains (wheat, spelt, kamut, farro, durum, semolina, bulgur, rye, triticale, non-gluten-free oats, beer)

Step Two

Over the next four days, record any symptoms you may be experiencing.

Experiencing any symptoms is a telltale sign that you are currently sensitive to the food in question and it is not benefiting you. It would be best to omit it from your diet. (You may, however, be able to successfully reintroduce the food again in the future, after further healing.)

If you do not experience a reaction to the food you've reintroduced after four days, you can add it back to your diet.

Step Three

Test the next food on the list.

Moving through the list in this way, you'll identify the foods you are sensitive to and are best avoided at this time to eliminate the frustrating symptoms that eating them causes you. You may decide that some foods should be gone from your diet for good, though you may find that with additional healing formerly inflammatory foods cause milder reactions or no reactions at all. As I've rebalanced my gut flora and resolved other root causes driving my symptoms, I've been able to reintroduce many foods that I was previously sensitive to, so that now I only avoid gluten and dairy. My diet has changed over time and yours will, too!

Use Your Symptoms to Determine Your Next Step

Symptoms	Solution
None! Adrenal symptoms have resolved.	Maintenance Protocol, page 258
Adrenal target symptoms remain: • Anxiety • Brain fog • Depression • Fatigue • Insomnia and sleep issues • Low libido • Pain	Advanced Stress Symptom Root Causes and Solutions, Chapter 10

Symptoms	Solution
Experiencing symptoms of toxicity: • Joint pain • Weight gain • Extreme sensitivity to supplements or medications • Chemical sensitivities • Night sweats • Skin breakouts, itchy skin, rashes, acne • Heat intolerance	Liver Support Protocol, found in my book *Hashimoto's Protocol*
Experiencing symptoms of gut imbalance: • Joint pain • Weight gain • Acid reflux • Bloating • Irritable bowel syndrome (IBS) • Stomach pain • You have been diagnosed with an autoimmune condition	Gut Balance Protocol, found in my book *Hashimoto's Protocol*

Advanced Adrenal Support: If You're Struggling with Adrenal Target Symptoms

You're feeling better but not yet 100 percent, as some symptoms of adrenal imbalance persist, such as anxiety, brain fog, depression, fatigue, insomnia and sleep issues, low libido, and pain. Please don't be discouraged! Some deeper healing may be all that you need to see more results. Here are three next steps for you to consider. You can choose to do one, two, or all three.

Next Step #1

Do the program for a little while longer. Don't be discouraged! It can take longer for some people to feel the full effects of the program, especially the diet and supplement components. Doing the program for a little while longer may move the needle on your lingering symptoms. Use the Maintenance Protocol (page 258) to help you. I also encourage you to implement any elements of the program you have not yet tried and that resonate with you now. I think you will see some additional success in doing this! Use the Fundamental Protocols of the ATP and the Symptom Relief They Support table below and the Adrenal Transformation Protocol Checklist (page 251) to help you identify interventions you may have missed.

The Fundamental Protocols of the ATP and the Symptom Relief They Support

This table is a quick summary of how the modalities can help with transforming your symptoms. I have put a plus in the categories that I have found to be especially helpful for a particular symptom through clinical experience and/or research.

Modality	Anxiety	Brain Fog	Fatigue	Mood	Libido	Sleep	Pain
Blood sugar balance	+	+	+	+	+	+	
Food sensitivities	+	+	+	+			+
Nutrient density	+	+	+	+	+	+	+
Hydration			+	+		+	
Caffeine reduction	+			+		+	
Adrenal support	+	+	+	+	+	+	+
Carnitine		+	+				+
Magnesium							+
Electrolytes		+	+			+	+
Myo-inositol	+				+	+	
Saccharomyces boulardii	+	+	+	+		+	
Mitochondrial support		+	+	+	+	+	+
Positive thought patterns	+		+	+			+
Pleasurable activities	+		+	+	+		+
Doing something creative	+	+	+	+	+		

Modality	Anxiety	Brain Fog	Fatigue	Mood	Libido	Sleep	Pain
Circadian rhythm	+		+	+	+	+	
Movement	+	+	+	+	+	+	+
Breathing	+	+	+	+	+	+	+
Healthy coping strategies	+	+	+	+	+	+	+
Letting go of the heaviness that weighs you down	+	+	+	+	+	+	+
Reclaiming your space	+	+	+	+	+	+	+

Next Step #2

Consult with a functional medicine practitioner. You may want to work with a knowledgeable functional medicine practitioner, who is well versed in addressing adrenal issues, to check your adrenals and identify which stage of adrenal dysfunction you are in. While the protocols in this program will benefit every stage and pattern of adrenal dysfunction, further testing may help identify additional, more specific interventions, such as hormones, medications, or supplements, based on your individualized hormone levels and patterns. See Adrenal Dysfunction Testing in the Advanced Stress Symptom Formulary (page 339) for more information.

Next Step #3

Check out the symptom-specific strategies in Chapter 10, "Advanced Stress Symptom Root Causes and Solutions" (page 267). Your body is telling us we should do some deeper digging to find the personal root causes driving your symptoms. We'll go symptom by symptom and identify ways to expand on the interventions already covered in the program as well as other potential root causes (and how to address them) and lab tests, lifestyle strategies, and supplements to consider. Start with the symptom that troubles you the most. Because the systems in our bodies are connected, addressing one symptom often leads to relief of other symptoms.

More Root Cause Digging: If You're Struggling with Other Symptoms

You've come a long way on your healing journey and are feeling noticeably better! Yet, you're struggling with additional deeper symptoms. While the ATP can address most symptoms of an impaired stress response, some symptoms may be rooted in other underlying issues. In many cases, these underlying issues are related to the liver and gut, and in my experience, people see the most improvements after implementing my Liver Support and Gut Balance protocols found in my book *Hashimoto's Protocol*. Many symptoms will often improve with liver and gut support, so you will likely see additional symptoms resolve by moving on to these as next steps. In some cases, addressing your symptoms may require professional healthcare support and advanced testing.

Next Step

Refer to Use Your Symptoms to Determine Your Next Step (page 261) for guidance.

Take the Next Step

No matter where you are on your healing journey, I hope you feel confident about your next steps and are empowered to continue taking control of your health and your life!

CHAPTER 10

Advanced Stress Symptom Root Causes and Solutions

We've come so far over the past few weeks. On the ATP, you've done a tremendous amount of work to heal your adrenals by sending your body safety signals through several healing modalities, such as balancing blood sugar, properly hydrating, and using supplements to support a healthy gut and mitochondria, to name just a few.

Each one of these interventions can help many of your symptoms, but if you've implemented the four-week ATP and are still struggling with anxiety, brain fog, depression, fatigue, sleep issues, low libido, and pain, there is still more we can do.

In this chapter, we'll go symptom by symptom to offer ways to dig deeper into the fundamental symptom-reduction strategies covered in the ATP and provide advanced healing modalities and protocols to consider based on potential root causes, including therapies, diets, devices, medications, and/or supplements as well as testing, where appropriate. Where indicated, more detailed information can be found in the Advanced Stress Symptom Formulary (page 339).

To get started, go to the table of contents on the following page and locate the remaining symptom you find the most frustrating, then turn to that section. If you have multiple symptoms, you may find that addressing one symptom helps relieve the others, but if not, turn to the root causes and solutions for each symptom as needed.

Advanced Stress Symptom Root Causes and Solutions Table of Contents

Brain Fog and Fatigue

I've combined these two symptoms because they share the same causes and solutions. You may have one or both symptoms. In my case, I started with fatigue and then progressed into brain fog.

Brain fog was one of the most personally devastating symptoms that I experienced due to adrenal and thyroid issues. As a person who had always excelled academically, I'd always prided myself on my brain's ability to recall important (and sometimes completely obscure) facts and details from experiences I'd had many years earlier. Fatigue was the second most devastating symptom, as it prevented me from achieving all of the things I wanted to achieve.

Many of the interventions we've been working on throughout the ATP may help reduce brain fog and fatigue, such as balancing blood sugar, eliminating inflammatory foods, and utilizing supplements to support mitochondrial function such as magnesium, carnitine, *Saccharomyces boulardii*, electrolytes with D-ribose, and adrenal adaptogens.

Additional ways to go deeper in the program to support brain fog and fatigue include:

- If you've done blood sugar balancing but are still experiencing fatigue, especially after meals, refer to Blood Sugar Support in the Advanced Stress Symptom Formulary (page 341) for additional strategies.
- Doing targeted food sensitivity testing can help you uncover the unique food triggers driving inflammation, often at the root of cloudy thinking and low energy. See Food Sensitivity Tests in Testing (page 368) for the tests I recommend.

- Drinking too much caffeine can create a vicious cycle of unrestful sleep followed by fatigue, leading to needing more caffeine and unrestful sleep, and on again. If you're currently drinking coffee, cocoa, soda, green tea, or black tea, removing or reducing your intake of caffeine can be helpful. (See What About Caffeine? on page 157 for more details.)

- A deficiency of B vitamins can contribute to a range of adrenal symptoms. The recommended adrenal support supplements contain a combination of B vitamins, but you may find additional stand-alone support of individual B vitamins, such as thiamine and B_6, beneficial. See Nutrients in the Advanced Stress Symptom Formulary (page 357) for more.

- If you have tried the circadian rhythm balancing and sleep hygiene strategies without success, consider adding blue light therapy to help regulate your sleep-wake cycles and review Insomnia and Sleep Issues in this chapter (page 273) for more potential root causes.

Other Potential Root Causes of Brain Fog and Fatigue
Thyroid hormone imbalance
Levels outside optimal ranges can lead to brain fog and fatigue. See Thyroid Hormones in the Advanced Stress Symptom Formulary (page 349) to learn more about how to optimize your thyroid levels.

Copper toxicity
Excess levels of copper can lead to fatigue and brain fog and should be investigated, especially if you have skin issues or poor wound healing. See Copper Toxicity in the Advanced Stress Symptom Formulary (page 352).

Environmental toxins
Various toxins, including heavy metals, can contribute to fatigue and cognitive difficulties. Consider liver support or testing for toxins (see Testing, page 371).

Gut imbalance/infections
An imbalance of gut bacteria or a gut infection may be at the root of your brain fog and anxiety. Many gut pathogens secrete neurotoxic substances,

including excess ammonia, that can lead to brain fog and fatigue, including *Helicobacter pylori, Clostridia, Candida,* and SIBO. Parasites like Giardia and *Blastocystis hominis* have also been implicated in brain fog and fatigue. Clearing infections will require interventions unique to each pathogen. A comprehensive stool analysis, SIBO breath test, and the Organic Acids Test can identify common triggering infections. Pathogen protocols can be found in my book *Hashimoto's Protocol* under Advanced Protocols.

Iron toxicity/overload

Excess iron is extremely toxic and may be at the root of fatigue and impaired cognitive function. For more, see Iron Toxicity/Overload in the Advanced Stress Symptom Formulary (page 356).

Low stomach acid and digestive enzymes

A lack of stomach acid and poor digestive function can contribute to poor cognitive function and low energy. Refer to Enzymes in the Advanced Stress Symptom Formulary (page 343) for more information and options.

Mitochondrial dysfunction

If mitochondria are damaged or functioning poorly, we'll struggle with tiredness and brain fog. Consider using the Organic Acids Test (page 371) to test for mitochondrial dysfunction and to determine further protocols.

Mold

If your symptoms started around the time that you moved into your home or office or after your home or office sustained water damage, there's a high likelihood that mold is at the root of your brain fog and fatigue. For ways to test for the presence of mold in your body and/or home, go to Testing for Mold (page 372).

Nutrient deficiencies

Riboflavin, thiamine, folate (vitamin B_9), iron, vitamin B_{12}, and vitamin D deficiencies can be at the root of brain fog and fatigue. See Nutrients in the Advanced Stress Symptom Formulary (page 357) for more guidance.

Reactivated Epstein-Barr (EBV)

The Epstein-Barr virus, the cause of mononucleosis, can persist in the host after the initial infection and can awaken and reactivate itself, even many years after its original activation. Symptoms include extreme fatigue, sore throat, rash, headache, and swollen tonsils and lymph nodes. Blood tests are used to figure out if a person has a reactivated infection. For more, see Epstein-Barr Reactivation in Testing (page 371).

Summary of Lab Tests to Consider for Brain Fog and Fatigue

- Comprehensive stool analysis
- Copper toxicity
- Food sensitivity testing
- Full thyroid panel
- Organic Acids Test
- Foundational nutrient panel
- Environmental toxin panel
- Mold mycotoxin panel
- Reactivated Epstein-Barr
- SIBO breath test

Interventions to Consider for Brain Fog and Fatigue

Reduce exposure to toxins

Reducing your exposure to toxins in your environment is especially important if you have unresolved fatigue. A few ideas include the use of an air purifier, drinking filtered water, stopping the use of cosmetics that contain petrochemicals, avoiding preservatives and additives, stopping the use of harsh cleaning agents and aerosols, and eliminating mold in your home. Taking 1,800 mg per day of N-acetyl-cysteine, a supplement that supports liver detox capabilities, may also be helpful.

Try a ketogenic diet

Some people find that eating a high-fat, low-carb ketogenic diet—where the body breaks down fats for fuel instead of relying on carbohydrates—can help stabilize blood sugar and keep insulin levels low, while providing your brain an alternate fuel source that also lowers inflammation. When done correctly, the ketogenic diet should give you more energy and awaken your brain. A common reason for feeling more tired includes deficiencies in digestive enzymes. See Enzymes in the Advanced Stress Symptom Formulary (page 343) for more.

Address sleep deprivation

Sleep deprivation can lead to brain fog and fatigue. If you are experiencing brain fog associated with sleep deprivation, try my Tired Mommy Protocol (also works for tired daddies and nonparents). ☺ These interventions are designed for maximizing quality of sleep and boosting energy levels throughout the day. If you are not breastfeeding, also see info on glycine in the Advanced Stress Symptom Formulary (page 360).

Always check with your doctor and watch your baby, but the following recommendations are generally considered to be safe for nursing moms and their nurslings.

- Getting lots of bright light in the morning.
- Grandparents—enough said!
- Carnitine, choline, omega-3s, and thiamine can help restore Mom's brain and energy levels from sleep deprivation and may also benefit nurslings (be sure to check with your pediatrician).
- B_{12} and ferritin are often depleted after giving birth and during lactation.
- Instead of the ABCs, consider gentle nursing-friendly adaptogens and a B Complex.
  - Reishi, Four Sigmatic Mushroom Hot Cacao with Reishi, one packet a day
  - Rhodiola is a gentle adaptogen that is generally considered safe for nursing mothers.
  - Tulsi tea is my go-to adaptogen during lactation. It also acts as a galactagogue and can help raise cortisol levels when needed. Organic India, one or two tea bags per day.
  - Shatavari, Organic India, one to two capsules, two times per day

- B-Complex Plus from Pure Encapsulations, one per day, or stand-alone B vitamins as needed (avoid B_6 > 50 mg)

Mitochondrial and sleep support
Coenzyme Q-10, copper, fulvic acid, manganese, N-acetyl-cysteine (NAC), omega-3 fatty acids, progesterone, selenium, vitamin D_3, vitamin E, and zinc are associated with improved energy production and brain function.

Neurotransmitters
People with brain fog and fatigue may benefit from the dopamine-boosting amino acid L-tyrosine and vitamin B_6. Please see *The Mood Cure* by Julia Ross for more guidance on using amino acids.

Nootropics
This broad range of drugs, supplements, and other substances, sometimes referred to as "smart drugs" or "cognitive enhancers," are taken to improve cognitive performance. I love benfotiamine, choline, glycine, lion's mane, L-tyrosine, omega-3 fatty acids, and trimethylglycine (TMG) for brain fog.

I would love to highlight benfotiamine, the fat-soluble version of thiamine (B_1), as an important nutrient to consider. After I published an article on using thiamine for fatigue, a reader wrote in who had been on disability, unable to work because of fatigue and brain fog for over ten years. She began taking a thiamine supplement. A few weeks after starting B_1, she was able to go back to work part-time, and eventually full-time, when her fatigue and brain fog lifted!

. . . .

See Nutrients (page 357) and Selected Herbs (page 366) in the Advanced Stress Symptom Formulary for more recommended products and dosages.

Insomnia and Sleep Issues
I've certainly dealt with my share of sleep challenges, both prior to my Hashimoto's diagnosis and more recently as a new mother. I know first-hand how important quality sleep is for my personal well-being—and as a

pharmacist working in functional medicine, the science is clear that sleep is fundamental to health and healing.

Many of the interventions we've been working on throughout the ATP should help improve your sleep cycle, including stabilizing blood sugar, maintaining proper hydration, rebalancing the circadian rhythm, releasing trauma, and supplementing with adaptogenic herbs, magnesium, and myo-inositol.

Additional ways to go deeper in the program to support sleep include:

- If you've done blood sugar balancing but are still experiencing night wakings between 2 and 3 a.m. that leave you anxious and needing a snack to go back to sleep, consider doing deeper work on your blood sugar balance. You may find that chromium can help with this (see Nutrients in the Advanced Stress Symptom Formulary, page 357). Refer to Blood Sugar Support in the Advanced Stress Symptom Formulary (page 341) for additional strategies.
- Try a different variety of caffeine-free relaxing tea (Balancing Teas, page 161) if you haven't yet found one that works for you.
- Caffeine wean. I used to consider myself to be a light sleeper . . . until I dropped my caffeine intake to two black teas each morning instead of having six to eight black teas a day (including my usual bedtime black tea). I was so surprised when things no longer woke me up at night!
- A deficiency of B vitamins can contribute to a range of adrenal symptoms. The recommended adrenal support supplements contain a combination of B vitamins, but you may find additional stand-alone support of individual B vitamins, such as thiamine and B_6, beneficial. See Nutrients in the Advanced Stress Symptom Formulary (page 357) for more.
- Switch your magnesium. Do note that the citrate version of magnesium may cause sleep issues in some (in others, glycinate may lead to sleep issues). For more information on magnesium and recommended brands, return to page 128.
- Insomnia and sleep issues, especially when associated with mood symptoms, can be due to trauma. Working with trauma-release therapies may be the path to resolving your sleep troubles.

Other Potential Root Causes of Insomnia and Sleep Issues

Copper toxicity

Excess copper can cause agitation, racing thoughts, restlessness, and insomnia. See Copper Toxicity in the Advanced Stress Symptom Formulary (page 352).

Flipped cortisol curve

Advanced adrenal testing can determine if elevated evening cortisol not responsive to the program interventions is an issue for you. See Adrenal Dysfunction Testing in the Advanced Stress Symptom Formulary (page 339).

Gut imbalance/infections

An imbalance of gut bacteria or a gut infection may be at the root of frequent night waking. Many gut pathogens secrete neurotoxic substances, including excess ammonia, that can lead to frequent night waking, including *H. pylori*. Ammonia can be cleared with ornithine to allow you to sleep well all night until infections are resolved. Clearing additional infections will require interventions unique to each pathogen. A comprehensive stool analysis, SIBO breath test, and the Organic Acids Test can identify common triggering infections. Pathogen protocols can be found in my book *Hashimoto's Protocol* under Advanced Protocols.

Hormonal imbalance

Estrogen dominance and/or low progesterone levels can be at the root of insomnia for some women, especially women over thirty-five. See Female Hormone Imbalance in the Advanced Stress Symptom Formulary (page 348) for more on rebalancing estrogen and progesterone.

Iron toxicity/overload

An excess of iron can lead to insomnia and troubled sleep. For more, see Iron Toxicity/Overload in the Advanced Stress Symptom Formulary (page 356).

Mold

Mold exposure and mycotoxins can lead to sleep issues and frequent night waking. For ways to test for the presence of mold in your body and/or home, go to Testing for Mold in Testing (page 372).

Nutrient deficiencies

Resolving deficiencies in folate (vitamin B_9), iron, vitamin B_{12}, and other vitamins can improve sleep. See Nutrients in the Advanced Stress Symptom Formulary (page 357) for more guidance.

Pyroluria

Pyroluria is linked to several sleep disorders. For more, see Pyroluria in the Advanced Stress Symptom Formulary (page 362).

Sleep apnea

Loud snoring, gasping for air during sleep, waking up with a sore throat or very dry mouth, morning headaches, restless sleep, and excessive daytime sleepiness are symptoms of sleep apnea, a chronic health condition often at the root of unrefreshing, fragmented sleep. If you're experiencing sleep issues and suspect you may have sleep apnea, speak with your practitioner, who may refer you to a sleep clinic. The standard of care for sleep apnea is the CPAP (continuous positive airway pressure) machine, and some have also reported benefits from using a mandibular advancement device. Please note that in some cases, sleep apnea may be due to a mitochondrial issue, and cases have reportedly been resolved with mitochondrial support, including high doses of thiamine. Reactivated EBV may play a role in sleep apnea. See Nutrients in the Advanced Stress Symptom Formulary (page 357) for more guidance.

Thyroid hormone imbalance

Insomnia and restlessness can be caused by an overactive thyroid due to Graves' disease or overmedication with thyroid hormones. See Thyroid Hormones in the Advanced Stress Symptom Formulary (page 349) to learn more about how to optimize your thyroid levels.

Summary of Lab Tests to Consider for Insomnia and Sleep Issues

- Adrenal dysfunction
- Comprehensive stool analysis
- Copper toxicity

- Female hormones
- Full thyroid panel
- Organic Acids Test
- Foundational nutrient panel
- Mold panel

Interventions to Consider for Insomnia and Sleep Issues
Neurotransmitters

Supporting mood-boosting neurotransmitters, such as dopamine (our "happy hormone") and serotonin (a stress-reducing hormone), promotes calmness and reduces tension and anxiety. I recommend 5HTP and GABA (gamma-aminobutyric acid). Please see *The Mood Cure* by Julia Ross for more guidance on using amino acids.

Sleep-supporting nutrients

To support more refreshing, deeper rest, consider supplementing with choline, glycine, and omega-3 fatty acids.

Melatonin

This sleep-cycle hormone can help you get back into your circadian rhythm routine by providing either an immediate release of melatonin for bedtime-only insomnia or melatonin in a delayed-release form to help with later-in-the-night awakenings. I recommend supplementing with Pure Encapsulations Melatonin or Herbatonin Plant Melatonin at bedtime, starting with the lowest dose and increasing until you find a dose between 0.5 and 5 mg that works for you.

Glycine

If you find that your sleep is not restful, you might want to try taking a glycine supplement at bedtime for more refreshing, deeper rest. A recent study found that glycine (a nonessential amino acid) subjectively and objectively improved sleep quality and reduced daytime sleepiness and fatigue in people with insomnia/sleep deprivation. Consider Designs for Health Glycine Powder at a dose of 3 grams per day.

....

See Nutrients (page 357) and Selected Herbs (page 366) in the Advanced Stress Symptom Formulary for more recommended products and dosages.

Low Libido

Many factors can lower one's libido, including something we've been talking a lot about on the ATP: chronic stress! All of our hormone systems are connected, so even a small change in one area can affect the others.

Coming back to the safety theory (discussed on page 15), our minds and bodies need to feel safe to enjoy sex, too. When adrenal dysfunction occurs, the body thinks it's in survival mode instead of thriving mode. Consequently, the adrenal glands can divert the production of "nice to have" hormones (like progesterone) from seemingly unneeded systems such as the body's reproductive system to fuel the production of hormones required for survival such as cortisol. This makes sense. If we're in survival mode, our bodies are too stressed out to worry about procreation, so no need for libido. Everything you've been doing to support your adrenals, including improving the quality of your sleep, boosting oxytocin, and decompressing with relaxing daily rituals, supports female hormone balance and libido, too. Libido is very connected to mood, sleep, pain, and energy levels, so sometimes the libido is the last thing that improves.

While it can be a difficult subject to discuss, please know that there are strategies you can consider to help improve your libido. If you feel that low libido is still a concern after you've completed the other protocols in this book, I encourage you to try a few new strategies.

Additional ways to go deeper in the program to resolve low libido include the following:

• Blood sugar swings can contribute to hormonal imbalances that can affect libido. If you've done blood sugar balancing but are still struggling with hormonal imbalances, refer to Blood Sugar Support in the Advanced Stress Symptom Formulary (page 341) for additional strategies.

- Inflammation is often at the root of pain, including pain related to the pelvic area that can contribute to low libido. Turn to Pain in this chapter (page 287) for more strategies to lower inflammation and relieve pain.
- A deficiency of B vitamins can contribute to a range of adrenal symptoms. The recommended adrenal support supplements contain a combination of B vitamins, but you may find additional stand-alone support of individual B vitamins, such as thiamine and B_6, beneficial. See Nutrients in the Advanced Stress Symptom Formulary (page 357) for more.
- Deficiencies in DHEA can contribute to low libido. DHEA can be boosted naturally with melatonin (getting lots of sleep), magnesium (supplements and Epsom salt baths), licorice, and meditation.
- Stress in interpersonal relationships and trauma can lead to libido issues. You may want to find a practitioner who can help you work through feelings and experiences that are making you feel unsafe and may be contributing to low libido.

Other Potential Root Causes of Low Libido
DHEA deficiency
DHEA levels decline with aging. In addition to the natural remedies for boosting DHEA, you may also wish to consider supplementing with low doses of DHEA. I prefer the topical DHEA-infused cream Julva, which can be used as a lubricant and is applied directly to the vulva, clitoris, and surrounding skin to help with vaginal rejuvenation, restoring moisture, preventing leaks, and improving sensation.

Please note that some individuals may over-convert DHEA into testosterone and estrogen, disrupting the balance of those two hormones. In some individuals, DHEA can also convert to androsterone and lead to symptoms such as acne, hair loss, mood swings, and facial hair (reishi and zinc may help balance this). Though DHEA is available without a prescription in the United States and a few other countries, I always recommend only using DHEA under the guidance of a practitioner, to find the right dosage for you. See Adrenal Dysfunction Testing in Testing (page 371) for the adrenal hormone tests I recommend.

Elevated prolactin

Breast tenderness, milky discharge from breasts outside of breastfeeding/pregnancy, enlarged breasts in males, libido issues, acne, excessive hair, infertility, and menstrual irregularities may all be clues that your prolactin is elevated. Elevated prolactin has been associated with autoimmune disease and HPA axis dysfunction. In some cases, elevated prolactin may be due to a small benign tumor on the pituitary gland, known as a prolactinoma. To normalize prolactin levels, consider:

Vitamin B$_6$, 150 mg twice daily (may shrink prolactinomas)
Chaste tree (Vitex), one capsule, twice daily
And in some cases, L-tyrosine, 500–1,500 mg, daily

Female hormone imbalance

Irregular periods, constant bloating, frequent mood fluctuations, heavy periods, brain fog, difficulty sleeping, and low libido are signs of female hormone imbalance. Female hormone imbalances, such as estrogen dominance and/or low progesterone, may lead to reduced desire. Testing hormone levels can be helpful and, in cases of low progesterone, supplementing with oral or topical bioidentical progesterone. See Female Hormones in Testing (page 371) for the tests I recommend and Female Hormone Imbalance in the Advanced Stress Symptom Formulary (page 348) for more.

Iron toxicity/overload

Too much iron may result in a decreased sex drive, especially in men. For more, see Iron Toxicity/Overload in the Formulary (page 356).

Low testosterone

Testosterone therapy is another potential treatment for women and can result in increased vaginal lubrication, heightened sexual arousal, and increased libido.

Medications

Antidepressants that are SSRIs (selective serotonin reuptake inhibitors) and birth control pills, among other medications, can lead to low libido. Discuss switching to a libido-boosting antidepressant such as bupropion with your doctor and consider nonhormonal alternatives to the birth control pill. See *Beyond the Pill* by Jolene Brighten.

Nutrient deficiencies
Nutrient deficiencies associated with low libido include iron (ferritin) and zinc. See Nutrients in the Advanced Stress Symptom Formulary (page 357).

PCOS
Many women with PCOS report low libido. Please see *Healing PCOS* by Amy Medling for more guidance.

Physical changes associated with menopause
If you are postmenopausal, in addition to the interventions in this book, you may wish to consider hormone therapies such as bioidentical hormones that can address symptoms such as hot flashes and vaginal dryness, which can impact libido.

Thyroid hormone imbalance
Thyroid hormone imbalances can throw off other hormones, as well as produce sexual dysfunction and low libido in both men and women. Restoring thyroid hormone levels can improve libido. See Thyroid Hormones in the Advanced Stress Symptom Formulary (page 349) to learn more about how to optimize your thyroid levels.

Summary of Lab Tests to Consider for Low Libido
- Full thyroid panel
- Nutrient panel
- Female hormones
- Mold panel
- Gut infection panel
- Functional medicine adrenal testing
- Adrenal hormones
- Prolactin

Interventions to Consider for Low Libido

Talk with your partner

It is important that they understand what is going on, that it can be improved upon, and that it isn't (or is) related to issues in your relationship.

Talk with your doctor

It is important that they know if you (or your partner) are experiencing low libido, as it can be a symptom of thyroid disease as well as other health issues, including chronic pain, depression, hypertension, diabetes, and cardiovascular disease.

Implement a seed rotation diet

Seed cycling is a method of balancing estrogen and progesterone.

- During the first half of the cycle (days 1 through 14), eat specific seeds to help the body produce estrogen: 2 tablespoons of fresh (not roasted) ground flax or pumpkin seeds per day.
- During the second half of the cycle (days 15 through 28), eat seeds that support progesterone production through zinc and vitamin E: 2 tablespoons of fresh (not roasted) ground sunflower seeds or sesame seeds per day.

This pattern can also be used by women in perimenopause or menopause to support hormone balance. You can prepare your own seeds, and I also like using the Beeya blend of nutrient-dense seeds in my salads and smoothies.

Chaste tree (Vitex)

Researchers believe that vitex works by decreasing levels of the hormone prolactin, which helps rebalance other hormones, including estrogen and progesterone. It's been shown to improve PMS symptoms, depression, anxiety, cravings, mood swings, headaches, and breast tenderness.

Maca

The Peruvian adaptogenic herb maca can help support your body's stress response and optimize adrenal health. It can also help improve libido and relieve menopause symptoms that might affect sexual desire, such as night sweats and hot flashes. I like the Femmenessence brand.

Shatavari
This is one of the most helpful adaptogens for libido.

Reduce inflammation with supplements
Consider adding N-acetyl-cysteine (NAC) and turmeric/curcumin to lower inflammation and help relieve pain, including vaginal and pelvic pain.

....

See Nutrients (page 357) and Selected Herbs (page 365) in the Advanced Stress Symptom Formulary for more recommended products and dosages.

Mood Disturbances: Anxiety, Depression, Overwhelm, Irritability, and Mood Swings

Mood instability, whether anxiety, depression, overwhelm, irritability, or mood swings, is a common symptom of adrenal dysfunction. I know how awful anxiety and overwhelm can feel, and feeling anxious perpetuates the vicious cycle of adrenal challenges.

On a grand scale, these symptoms, just like most other symptoms we experience, are a sign that something is out of balance within our bodies or our lives. In my experience, mood can often be stabilized with blood sugar balance, addressing nutrient deficiency/excess, targeting inflammation, and/ or focusing on hormonal imbalance.

We address the most common reasons for mood issues in the ATP, and so most people following the full program do report a marked reduction in mood-related symptoms over the four weeks.

NOTE: If you are currently taking prescription antidepressants or antianxiety medications, do not stop taking your medications without the oversight of your physician or therapist.

Additional ways to go deeper in the program to support mood include:

- If you've done blood sugar balancing but are still experiencing mood swings, anxiety, and/or hanger, refer to Blood Sugar Support in the

Advanced Stress Symptom Formulary (page 341) for additional strategies. L-glutamine and Amino-NR may be helpful for anxiety due to blood sugar issues.

- Inflammatory foods can contribute to mood imbalance. One type of food to consider eliminating right away if you have anxiety is nuts. I am not 100 percent sure what it is about nuts that causes this reaction (it could be high copper content, high omega-6, oxalate content, or fat malabsorption), but I have seen numerous clients experience mood reactions with nuts, especially with almonds. Consider an elimination diet or food sensitivity testing to uncover offending foods.
- If you're currently drinking caffeinated beverages, including coffee, soda, green tea, or black tea, removing or reducing your intake of caffeine can be helpful with anxiety, mood swings, and irritability. Some people may even react to cocoa.
- A deficiency of B vitamins can contribute to a range of adrenal symptoms. The recommended adrenal support supplements contain a combination of B vitamins, but you may find additional stand-alone support of individual B vitamins, such as thiamine and B_6, beneficial. See Nutrients in the Advanced Stress Symptom Formulary (page 357) for more.
- Consider adding blue light therapy to your circadian rhythm–balancing strategies if you haven't already. It can help with seasonal affective disorder (SAD) as well as generally supporting a more positive mood and easing depression.
- We talked about the healing power of creating. If you love art, you may want to go deeper and work with a trained therapist on art therapy, which has been found to significantly reduce trauma symptoms and decrease levels of depression in adults who experienced trauma.

Other Potential Root Causes of Mood Disturbances
Copper toxicity
A toxic buildup of copper may be at the root of anxiety, racing thoughts, mood swings, fatigue, and insomnia. For more, see Copper Toxicity in the Advanced Stress Symptom Formulary (page 352).

Female hormone imbalances

Estrogen dominance and/or low progesterone may lead to many symptoms like irritability, mood lability, depression, and mood swings. Testing hormone levels can be helpful. If tests reveal low progesterone, supplementing with oral or topical bioidentical progesterone might just be the chill pill you need. See Female Hormones in Testing (page 371) for the tests I recommend and Female Hormone Imbalance in the Advanced Stress Symptom Formulary (page 348) for more.

Gut imbalance/infection

An imbalance of gut bacteria as well as various infections can contribute to mood issues; most notably an overgrowth of *Clostridia* and yeast in the gut has been associated with mood-related conditions as diverse as autism, depression, anxiety, mood swings, and schizophrenia. An overgrowth of *Streptococcus* has been associated with obsessive-compulsive disorder. Consider using the Organic Acids Test to find whether *Clostridia* or yeast is an issue for you, or a gut health test like the GI-MAP to find whether *Streptococcus* could be behind your symptoms.

Iron toxicity/overload

A buildup of too much iron can cause irritability and depression. For more, see Iron Toxicity/Overload in the Advanced Stress Symptom Formulary (page 356).

Mold

There is a big connection between mood issues and mold exposure. For ways to test for the presence of mold in your body and/or home, go to Testing for Mold in Testing (page 372).

Nutrient deficiencies

Addressing the following nutrient depletions can be a genuine game changer when it comes to improving mood: omega-3 fatty acids, folate (vitamin B_9), iron, vitamin B_{12}, and vitamin D. See Nutrients in the Advanced Stress Symptom Formulary (page 357) for testing and more.

Pyroluria

Symptoms of social anxiety have been associated with pyroluria. For more, see Pyroluria in the Advanced Stress Symptom Formulary (page 361).

Thyroid hormone imbalance

Levels outside optimal ranges can cause anxiety, depression, and irritability. See Thyroid Hormones in the Advanced Stress Symptom Formulary (page 349) to learn more about how to optimize your thyroid levels.

Lab Tests to Consider for Mood Disturbances

- Full thyroid panel
- Copper toxicity
- Food sensitivity testing
- Nutrient panel
- Female hormones
- Mold panel
- Gut infection panel
- Organic Acids Test (gut infections)
- Functional medicine adrenal testing
- Adrenal hormones
- Prolactin
- Pyroluria

Interventions to Consider for Mood Disturbances

Targeted homeopathy

Bach Flower remedies are a type of homeopathic medicine. Try Bach Rescue Remedy, a blend of flowers known to help calm the nerves.

Yoga

Gentle forms of yoga, such as hatha and yin, have been shown to calm the nervous system, relax the mind, and relieve symptoms of depression.

Neurotransmitters

People with anxiety, depression, mood swings, and other mood imbalances often experience a deficiency in their mood-boosting neurotransmitters, such as dopamine (our "happy" hormone) and serotonin (a stress-reducing hormone). Supplements that support the production of neurotransmitters can be helpful and include 5HTP, GABA (gamma-aminobutyric acid), L-tyrosine, and vitamin B$_6$. Please see *The Mood Cure* by Julia Ross for more guidance on using amino acids.

Nutritional lithium (lithium orotate)

An essential micronutrient with a long history of clinical use for supporting healthy mood and behavior by promoting the activity of dopamine and serotonin. May be especially helpful for irritability.

Address OCD

If testing your gut revealed an overgrowth of *Streptococcus,* consider the herb berberine, to help with rebalancing this bacteria, which can often resolve obsessive symptoms. Additional options for OCD include increasing myoinositol (doses as high as 18 grams per day have been used for OCD). A starting dose may be 3 grams per day in three divided doses. Additionally, NAC can be helpful for some individuals.

Omega-3 fatty acids and zinc

Both help support mood by lowering inflammation.

....

See Nutrients (page 357) and Selected Herbs (page 365) in the Advanced Stress Symptom Formulary for recommended products and dosages.

Pain

As a pharmacist, I certainly understand the value of pain medication and other conventional therapies in the right context. However, I also know that getting to the root cause of why we have pain and treating the trigger itself—often through natural methods—can be more effective at providing a long-term resolution to pain—without many of the unwanted side effects associated with conventional approaches. Inflammation is often at the root when it comes to pain, and several natural approaches have been shown to be effective at targeting the cause of the inflammation, thus reducing inflammation and pain while promoting healing.

Wherever you are on your healing journey, I want you to be encouraged that you are not limited to a life of pain, nor are you required to suffer the side effects of addictive medications. There are many natural solutions to pain management that can help you feel better and live your life.

Many of the interventions we've been working on throughout the ATP are designed to lower inflammation and ease pain, such as balancing blood sugar, removing reactive foods, supporting with magnesium and B vitamins, and boosting oxytocin.

Additional ways to go deeper in the program to reduce pain include:

- If you've done blood sugar balancing but are still experiencing blood sugar swings and hanger, refer to Blood Sugar Support in the Advanced Stress Symptom Formulary (page 341) for additional strategies.
- A deficiency of B vitamins can contribute to a range of adrenal symptoms. The recommended adrenal support supplements contain a combination of B vitamins, but you may find additional stand-alone support of individual B vitamins, such as thiamine and B_6, beneficial. See Nutrients in the Advanced Stress Symptom Formulary (page 357) for more.
- A beneficial form of healing touch to boost oxytocin, massage is good for your mood and pain relief. Consider other forms of therapeutic bodywork found to be helpful with pain such as chiropractic care, rolfing (a form of holistic bodywork that uses hands-on manipulation of the body's soft tissue to create balance and alignment in the body), physical therapy, osteopathic manipulative treatment (a practitioner uses stretches, gentle pressure, and resistance to move a patient's muscles and joints), and craniosacral therapy (uses gentle pressure to manipulate the joints in the cranium or skull, parts of the pelvis, and the spine).

Other Potential Root Causes of Pain

Gut imbalance/infections

An imbalance of gut bacteria or a gut infection may be at the root of your pain. *Klebsiella, Proteus,* and *Citrobacter* are some potential pathogens associated with pain. Clearing infections will require interventions unique to each pathogen. A comprehensive stool analysis, SIBO breath test, and the Organic Acids Test can identify common triggering infections. Pathogen protocols can be found in my book *Hashimoto's Protocol* under Advanced Protocols.

Inflammatory foods

Reactive foods can contribute to pain. Here are a few common pain-inducing food groups to consider eliminating for two weeks to determine if they are reactive for you:

- Oxalates
- FODMAPS
- Nightshades (including the adaptogen ashwagandha)
- Salicylates

Doing targeted food sensitivity testing can help you uncover the unique food triggers causing chronic inflammation. See Food Sensitivity Testing in Testing (page 371) for the tests I recommend.

Iron toxicity/overload

Stomach and joint pain are two early symptoms of too much iron. For more, see Iron Toxicity/Overload in the Advanced Stress Symptom Formulary (page 356).

Thyroid hormone imbalance

Hypothyroidism and hyperthyroidism have been associated with pain. See Thyroid Hormones in the Advanced Stress Symptom Formulary (page 349) to learn more about how to optimize your thyroid levels.

Summary of Lab Tests to Consider for Pain

- Comprehensive stool analysis
- Food sensitivity testing

- Foundational nutrient panel
- Organic Acids Test
- SIBO breath test
- Full thyroid panel

Interventions to Consider for Pain

A healing diet

For certain kinds of pain, the ketogenic diet can be helpful. For other types of pain, the Low FODMAPs Diet, Autoimmune Paleo Diet, and low oxalate diet are associated with pain relief.

Acupuncture

The research supports the use of acupuncture for pain relief, and it is becoming more and more common in the West as an alternative to habit-forming opiates. Results from several studies suggest that acupuncture may help ease chronic pain, such as low-back pain, neck pain, and osteoarthritis pain. It has also been shown to reduce the frequency of tension headaches and prevent migraine headaches.

Cold laser therapy

Also known as low-level laser therapy (LLLT), cold laser therapy utilizes specific wavelengths of light to interact with tissue, in order to help accelerate the healing process, which can help eliminate pain and inflammation.

Investigate platelet-rich plasma injections (PRP)

PRP therapy has emerged in recent years as a promising treatment for chronic pain, and has even been used postsurgery to speed up the healing process. PRP may benefit those with arthritis, sciatic pain, tendonitis, carpal tunnel, and musculoskeletal pain.

B vitamins

Thiamine (vitamin B_1) at high doses of 600 to 1,800 mg/day can help with pain from fibromyalgia, and vitamin B_6 taken at a dose of 100 to 200 mg/day can relieve carpal tunnel syndrome.

Neurotransmitters

GABA, which supports the production of GABA (our "chill" neurotransmitter that helps with muscle relaxation), and 5HTP, which supports serotonin production, are both helpful for pain. (Low serotonin has been a long-known potential target for pain relief and pharmaceutical agents, including SSRIs like Paxil.) Please see *The Mood Cure* by Julia Ross for more guidance on using neurotransmitters.

Omega-3 fatty acids

Omega-3s are a powerful ally against pain, helping to lower the oxidative stress contributing to chronic inflammation.

Systemic enzymes

Systemic enzymes have been shown to be as effective for pain as the NSAID diclofenac for painful knee arthritis, but with far fewer side effects.

Trimethylglycine (TMG)

Trimethylglycine (TMG) helps break down protein, thereby aiding digestion and reducing intestinal inflammation. It can also be helpful for breaking down homocysteine, which has been associated with inflammation. Furthermore, it can increase the amount of SAMe, a naturally occurring substance with mood-boosting and pain-relieving properties, within the body.

Turmeric

Curcumin, the active component in turmeric, has been found to have therapeutic anti-inflammatory effects for a variety of gastrointestinal conditions, including Crohn's disease, ulcerative colitis, and irritable bowel syndrome, and to reduce joint inflammation in rheumatoid arthritis.

....

See Nutrients (page 357) and Selected Herbs (page 365) in the Advanced Stress Symptom Formulary for more recommended products and dosages.

To view the scientific references cited in this chapter, please visit us online at https://thyroidpharmacist.com/atpbooknotes.

Author's Note

It is my sincere hope that you're feeling lighter, brighter, and less stressed! With the fundamental protocols of the ATP and the additional strategies in Part III (if you needed them), you've sent your body an abundance of safety signals to promote rest and healing. Celebrate your success! And don't be discouraged if more healing is needed in order for all of your symptoms to vanish. It may just take a little more digging into your unique root causes—and patience!—for your symptoms to resolve. I want you to know that I'm here for you as you take the next steps to transform your health and feel like yourself again.

I am honored that you have entrusted me with your health and allowed me to be a part of your journey. I hope we will stay connected through my website and social media. I love hearing feedback from my community and sharing the latest research and solutions for reversing adrenal imbalance and Hashimoto's as well as offering an abundance of support. I wish you continued success on your healing journey!

Izabella Wentz, PharmD, FASCP
www.ThyroidPharmacist.com
www.facebook.com/ThyroidLifestyle
@IzabellaWentzPharmD

Recipes

Sides

Snacks

Drinks

ADRENAL KICK START
Serves 1

The Adrenal Kick Start utilizes vitamin C–rich orange juice and sea salts/electrolytes to raise your morning blood glucose and cortisol levels, but couples them with fat and protein to ensure a smooth level of energy throughout the day. As a bonus, it tastes like an orange Creamsicle.

½ cup freshly squeezed orange juice

¼ cup full-fat canned coconut milk

½ serving of Rootcology protein powder of choice (or other compliant protein powder)

¼ to ½ teaspoon sea salt or pink Himalayan sea salt to taste

In a blender, blend the orange juice, coconut milk, protein powder, and salt until smooth and frothy.

Notes

Start with ¼ teaspoon of sea salt. If you feel you need more, then add up to another ¼ teaspoon of sea salt.

Although orange juice is high in sugar, the oxytocin-releasing fats and clean protein help counterbalance the sugar rush that one would typically get with drinking just orange juice. The orange juice is also a great source of vitamin C (one of the ABCs of adrenal support).

For those who are sensitive to citrus, the orange juice can be substituted with one of the alternate vitamin C–rich juices or fruits below:

½ cup tart cherry juice (found in most health food/grocery stores—ensure it does not contain added sugar)

½ cup acerola cherry juice (may be difficult to source)

⅓ cup organic strawberries (blended with ¼ cup of water)

1 organic kiwi (blended with ¼ cup of water)

KETO-FRIENDLY ADRENAL KICK START OPTIONS

I've created a few variations of the Adrenal Kick Start that are compliant with ketogenic diets, should you be following one.

Adrenal Kick Start—Keto Version #1
Serves 1

1 serving of flavored electrolytes like Rootcology Electrolyte Blend* or Designs for Health Electrolyte Synergy

½ cup water

¼ cup full-fat canned coconut milk

½ serving of Rootcology protein powder of choice (or other compliant protein powder)

¼ to ½ teaspoon sea salt

In the bowl of a blender, blend the electrolyte blend, water, coconut milk, protein powder, and sea salt until smooth and frothy.

This will satisfy your electrolyte needs for the day, so no need to consume additional electrolyte supplements.

Adrenal Kick Start—Keto Version #2
Serves 1

1 teaspoon camu camu powder

½ cup water

¼ cup full-fat canned coconut milk

½ serving of Rootcology protein powder of choice (or other compliant protein powder)

In a blender, blend the camu camu powder, water, coconut milk, and protein powder until smooth and frothy.

FAT GREEN JUICE
Serves 1

Packed with easy-to-digest nutrients and energy-boosting fats, this green juice is a tasty and satisfying mid-morning or mid-afternoon snack.

6 or 7 baby carrots
1 Granny Smith apple
3 or 4 celery stalks
1 small cucumber
3 cups finely chopped kale
1 organic lime, peeled
1 tablespoon coconut oil or MCT oil, melted
Sea salt or pink Himalayan salt to taste

1. In a juicer, juice the carrots, apple, celery, cucumber, kale, and lime.
2. Once juiced, add the melted oil and sea salt and stir to combine.

Notes
If you don't have a juicer, blend the ingredients, except for the oil and salt, with 1 to 2 cups of filtered water. Then push and strain through a fine-mesh sieve or nut milk bag. Stir in the oil and salt.

Please be aware that if you have never used MCT oil (medium-chain triglycerides) before, but are interested, you will want to start slow. MCT oil can have a laxative effect, and #disasterpants is not something that we want you to experience throughout the ATP! To incorporate MCT oil, start with ¼ teaspoon, then slowly increase the amount over time by ¼ teaspoon, until you reach your desired threshold of MCT oil.

MACA LATTE
Serves 1

A warming maca latte laced with blood sugar–balancing cinnamon is a great way to start the day—especially when you're trying to wean off caffeine. One of my favorite adaptogens, maca can help improve energy, mood, and sexual desire. No wonder this beverage has earned the nickname "Hello, libido" latte!

1 tablespoon maca powder
1 tablespoon full-fat canned coconut milk
1 teaspoon ground cinnamon, plus more for garnish (optional)
1 cup hot water
Stevia to taste (optional)

1. Blend the maca, coconut milk, cinnamon, hot water, and stevia (if using) together in a blender.
2. Top with some extra cinnamon if desired.

Note
Maca is an adaptogen and can help stabilize the adrenals. However, it may have different effects for different people. So it may be best to start with 1 teaspoon to determine how you tolerate it, and then work your way up to the recommended 1 tablespoon.

SPA WATER
Serves 8

If you've gotten bored of plain water, kick the flavor up a notch by adding fruit, vegetables, and herbs. Spa robe not required. ☺

1 pitcher of filtered water

1 cup chopped (½-inch) or sliced (¼-inch) fruit and/or vegetables

Fresh herb(s) of choice

For the blends, you can use whatever combination you like, equaling 1 cup of fruit and/or vegetables, so long as the foods are compliant—here are a few of my favorites:

Blend 1: Strawberry, cucumber, and mint

Blend 2: Lemon and lime

Blend 3: Basil and orange

1. Cut pieces of fruit/vegetables/herbs of your choice.
2. Place all of the ingredients in the large pitcher of water.
3. Sip throughout the day.

SOLE

Makes 3 cups of concentrate

Sole is a hydrating, high-concentration mixture of salt and filtered water. High-quality, minimally processed sea salt provides electrolyte-rich sodium and trace minerals.

1 cup Himalayan or Celtic sea, plus more as needed

1 large Mason jar with lid

3 cups filtered water

1. Add the salt to the Mason jar, and then fill the rest of the jar with filtered water.
2. Put the lid on the jar and shake gently; leave overnight.
3. If there is some salt left in the jar, the sole is ready to use. If there is no salt left in the jar, add some more salt, ¼ cup at a time, and let it dissolve. Keep adding ¼ cup of salt until there is some sediment at the bottom of the jar.

4. When ready to use, add 1 teaspoon of sole to a glass of water, and drink it on an empty stomach, 30 to 60 minutes away from thyroid medications.
5. If detox reactions occur, start with ¼ teaspoon and work your way up to 1 teaspoon.

Notes

Store at room temperature. This mixture will last indefinitely due to the antimicrobial and antifungal properties of the salt. Do not use metal utensils to measure the sole, as the salt can react with the metals.

Please be sure to speak with a practitioner if you have any concerns about consuming added salt.

TULSI TEA LATTE

Serves 1

This is my go-to beverage when I need a delicious way to relax and unwind. The adaptogen tulsi works wonders on mood and overall stress levels, while good fats and protein make this a rich, satisfying drink—and a blood sugar–balanced one.

1 bag tulsi tea with rose
1 cup hot filtered water
2 tablespoons full-fat canned coconut milk
1 teaspoon ground cinnamon
1 scoop collagen protein
Pinch of sea salt or pink Himalayan salt
Stevia to taste (optional)

1. Prepare the tulsi tea with hot water and let it steep for 3 to 5 minutes, then remove the tea bag.
2. In the bowl of a blender, add the coconut milk, cinnamon, collagen protein, salt, and stevia (if using), along with the steeped tulsi tea.
3. Blend until all ingredients are thoroughly mixed.

Smoothies

ADRENAL TONIC SMOOTHIE

Serves 1

In this refreshing smoothie, an orange supplies a rich source of adrenal-healing vitamin C and easy-to-digest fiber, while the fat from the coconut milk alongside the protein powder helps prevent blood sugar swings. Adding electrolyte-rich coconut water and salt creates a powerfully hydrating beverage.

½ cup coconut water

¼ cup full-fat canned coconut milk

1 small organic orange, peeled and chopped

1 very small cucumber

1 medium carrot

½ teaspoon alcohol-free vanilla extract or vanilla beans

Stevia to taste (optional)

¼ teaspoon sea salt or pink Himalayan salt

1 serving of Rootcology protein powder of choice (or other compliant protein powder)

In the bowl of a high-speed blender, such as a Vitamix, blend the coconut water, coconut milk, orange, cucumber, carrot, vanilla, stevia (if using), salt, and protein powder until a smooth consistency is achieved.

BLUEBERRY PIE SMOOTHIE

Serves 1

Combining blueberries—blood sugar–balancing and antioxidant powerhouses—with satiating good fats and protein, fiber- and nutrient-rich leafy greens, hydrating coconut water and salt, and a touch of warming cinnamon and vanilla, my Blueberry Pie Smoothie elevates the delicious, adrenal-supporting ingredients of one of my favorite desserts into a richly satisfying and healing smoothie perfect for breakfast or an anytime snack.

½ cup full-fat canned coconut milk

¼ cup coconut water

½ cup organic blueberries

1 handful of baby spinach

1 very small cucumber

Pinch of sea salt

Pinch of ground cinnamon

½ teaspoon alcohol-free vanilla extract or vanilla beans

Stevia to taste (optional)

1 serving of Rootcology protein powder of choice (or other compliant protein powder)

In the bowl of a high-speed blender, such as a Vitamix, blend the coconut milk, coconut water, blueberries, spinach, cucumber, salt, cinnamon, vanilla, stevia (if using), and protein powder until a smooth consistency is achieved.

ROOT CAUSE GREEN SMOOTHIE
Serves 1

Packed with nutrition for your adrenals, the Root Cause Green Smoothie helps balance blood sugar and reduce inflammation thanks to the good fats in the avocado and coconut milk. It makes for an energizing breakfast every morning!

½ cup mixed baby greens

1 small carrot

⅓ ripe avocado

½ celery stalk

1 cucumber

2 tablespoons fresh basil

⅔ cup full-fat canned coconut milk

1 scoop of Rootcology protein powder of choice (or other compliant protein powder)

In the bowl of a high-speed blender, such as a Vitamix, blend the baby greens, carrot, avocado, celery, cucumber, basil, coconut milk, and protein powder until a smooth consistency is achieved.

Soups/Salads

EVERYDAY DRESSING
Makes ½ cup

This super simple yet flavorful dressing is rich in healthy fats and a dose of vitamin C to drizzle over salads, roasted vegetables, or anything at all!

¼ cup extra-virgin olive oil

¼ cup freshly squeezed lemon juice

1 tablespoon dried basil (or other dried herbs of choice)

1. In a small bowl, mix the olive oil, lemon juice, and dried basil.
2. Refrigerate until ready to serve.

BONE BROTH
Makes 8 servings

Bone broth is a nutrient-dense, hydrating food that contains an abundance of gut-healing minerals and amino acids. I like to make a large batch and freeze the excess in single-serve containers (it keeps for up to three months in the freezer) so I always have some on hand for a warming drink or to use in soups and stews.

4 or 5 chicken legs

1 tablespoon apple cider vinegar

2 stalks celery

1 onion

6 to 8 large carrots

Purified water

Sea salt or pink Himalayan salt to taste

Freshly ground black pepper to taste (if tolerated)

Slow Cooker Directions:

1. Place the chicken, vinegar, and vegetables in a slow cooker.
2. Fill with water, cover, and cook on high for 8 to 12 hours.
3. Season with salt and pepper (if tolerated) to taste.
4. Strain, pour it into Mason jars, and refrigerate. Remove solidified fat before using or freezing.

Stovetop Directions:

1. Place the chicken, vinegar, and vegetables in a stockpot.
2. Fill with purified water.
3. Bring to a boil over high heat, reduce the heat to medium-low, and simmer for 8 to 12 hours.
4. Season with salt and pepper (if tolerated) to taste.
5. Strain, pour into Mason jars, and refrigerate. Remove solidified fat before using or freezing.

Electric Pressure Cooker Directions:

1. Place the chicken, vinegar, and vegetables in the pot of the pressure cooker.
2. Fill two-thirds of the way up with purified water.
3. Press the "Manual" button, set the pressure to high, and set the timer to 90 minutes.
4. Season with salt and pepper (if tolerated) to taste.
5. Strain, pour into Mason jars, and refrigerate. Remove solidified fat before using or freezing.

COCONUT BASIL & BEEF SOUP
Serves 4

This flavorful Thai-inspired soup brightens any weekday! Cauliflower provides plenty of fiber and vitamin C, and the coconut milk creates a luscious creamy base, full of beneficial fats.

1 tablespoon extra-virgin olive oil

2 garlic cloves, minced

1 pound ground beef

1 large head of cauliflower, cut into florets

4 cups bone broth (store-bought, or see recipe on page 305)

1 (14-ounce) can full-fat coconut milk

1 cup chopped celery

¼ cup chopped fresh basil

Sea salt or pink Himalayan salt to taste

Freshly ground black pepper to taste (if tolerated)

1. In a large pot over medium heat, heat the olive oil.
2. Add the garlic to the pot. Cook for 2 minutes, then add the beef and cauliflower. Cook for 5 minutes, until the beef is browned.
3. Add the bone broth, coconut milk, celery, basil, salt, and pepper (if tolerated) to the pot and stir.
4. Cover and reduce the heat to low. Simmer for 20 minutes, until the beef is cooked through and the vegetables are tender.
5. Serve warm.

LEEK & SPINACH TURKEY SOUP
Serves 4

Leek & Spinach Turkey Soup is perfect on a chilly day or any day when you want the healing benefits of a simple, tasty soup. Spinach, one of my favorite leafy greens, is rich in iron, vitamin C, potassium, and magnesium, while leeks, a rich source of antioxidants, add a sweeter, more delicate oniony flavor to gut-healing, nutrient-dense bone broth.

¼ cup coconut oil

1 large leek, diced

4 cups bone broth (store-bought, or see recipe on page 305)

3 cups ground turkey, browned

Sea salt or pink Himalayan salt to taste

Freshly ground black pepper to taste (if tolerated)

1 teaspoon ground sage

4 cups spinach

1. In a large pot, heat 2 tablespoons of the coconut oil over medium heat. Add the leek and sauté for 5 minutes.
2. Add the remaining 2 tablespoons of the coconut oil, and then add the bone broth, ground turkey, salt, pepper (if tolerated), and sage. Raise the heat to high and bring the soup to a boil.
3. Reduce the heat to low and cover the pot. Simmer the soup for 30 minutes, until the vegetables are slightly tender.
4. Once the soup is done, remove the pot from the heat and stir in the spinach until wilted.
5. Serve warm.

MEATBALL & MUSHROOM SOUP

Serves 4

This hearty soup is a nutritional powerhouse, loaded with ingredients that provide a wide variety of vitamins and minerals, such as iron, B vitamins, vitamin C, and magnesium, and fiber. Garnish with green onion for an added punch of anti-inflammatory antioxidants!

1 pound ground beef

2 tablespoons coconut flour

Sea salt or pink Himalayan salt to taste

Freshly ground black pepper to taste (if tolerated)

½ teaspoon dried thyme

½ tablespoon coconut oil

2 cups sliced mushrooms

1 large stalk celery, chopped

1 cup cauliflower florets

¼ cup chopped green onion, plus more for garnish

4 cups bone broth (store-bought, or see recipe on page 305)

1 (14-ounce) can full-fat coconut milk

2 cups baby spinach, chopped

1. In a large bowl, mix the beef, flour, salt, pepper (if tolerated), and thyme. Form the meat mixture into meatballs.
2. In a large pot over medium heat, heat the coconut oil. Add the meatballs and cook on each side for 2 minutes, until browned.
3. Add the mushrooms, celery, cauliflower, and green onions. Continue to sauté until the vegetables start to get tender and brown slightly.
4. Add the bone broth and coconut milk and bring to a boil, then reduce the heat to a simmer over medium heat.
5. Simmer for another 20 minutes, until the meatballs are no longer pink in the center and the vegetables are tender.
6. Remove from the heat and add the chopped spinach; mix until wilted.
7. Garnish with the reserved green onion and serve warm.

KALE & CUCUMBER CHICKEN SALAD
Serves 4

A healthy spin on traditional chicken salad, Kale & Cucumber Chicken Salad uses a hint of coconut milk to add creaminess instead of mayonnaise, and cucumber adds crunch and promotes adequate hydration. High in vitamins A and C, calcium, magnesium, and B vitamins, kale has earned its place as one of the most nutrient-dense foods on the planet. Chilling the salad or giving it time to rest at room temperature before serving helps tenderize the kale and marry the flavors.

½ pound ground chicken, cooked

2 cups kale, chopped

2 tablespoons fresh parsley, chopped

2 cups cucumber, chopped

¼ cup freshly squeezed lemon juice

2 teaspoons apple cider vinegar

2 tablespoons canned full-fat coconut milk

1 tablespoon coconut oil, melted

¼ cup chopped red onion

Sea salt or pink Himalayan salt to taste

Freshly ground black pepper to taste (if tolerated)

1. In a large bowl, mix the chicken, kale, parsley, and cucumbers together.
2. In a small bowl, whisk the lemon juice, vinegar, coconut milk, coconut oil, red onion, salt, and pepper (if tolerated) to create the dressing.
3. Pour the dressing over the salad and toss.
4. Serve chilled or at room temperature.

SALMON & BRUSSELS SPROUT SALAD
Serves 4

This light, bright salad is bursting with flavor and digestive support thanks to lemon juice and dill. Salmon is high in omega-3 fatty acids and a great source of protein, and Brussels sprouts are a good source of vitamin C and folate.

2 cups shredded Brussels sprouts

2 cups salmon, cooked and flaked

2 tablespoons freshly squeezed lemon juice

2 tablespoons extra-virgin olive oil

1 tablespoon minced fresh dill, or 1 teaspoon dried dill

1 small shallot, minced

Sea salt or pink Himalayan salt to taste

Freshly ground black pepper to taste (if tolerated)

In a large bowl, mix the Brussels sprouts, salmon, lemon juice, olive oil, dill, shallot, salt, and pepper (if tolerated). Serve immediately.

Dinner

BUTTERNUT SPAGHETTI & TURKEY MEATBALLS
Serves 4

Try this when you're craving spaghetti and meatballs—but not the blood sugar crash and food coma the traditional dish can cause! Coconut aminos, made from the sap of coconut trees, help support a healthy gut and mood. Replace the spiralized butternut squash with spiralized zucchini to change it up!

1 pound ground turkey

Sea salt or pink Himalayan salt to taste

Freshly ground black pepper to taste (if tolerated)

½ teaspoon fresh cilantro or parsley, chopped

1 small onion, finely chopped

1 teaspoon freshly squeezed lime juice

1 tablespoon fresh sage, minced

¼ cup coconut oil

¼ cup coconut aminos

1 large butternut squash, peeled, seeded, and spiralized

1. In a large bowl, mix the turkey, salt, pepper (if tolerated), cilantro, onion, lime juice, and sage together. Form the meat mixture into meatballs.
2. In a large skillet over medium heat, heat 2 tablespoons of the coconut oil. Add the meatballs to the oil and cook on each side for 2 minutes, until browned.
3. Pour the coconut aminos over the meatballs. Cover and reduce the heat to low. Simmer for 10 minutes, until the meatballs are no longer pink in the center.

4. In a separate pan, heat the remaining 2 tablespoons of coconut oil and stir-fry the spiralized butternut squash noodles for 3 minutes, until cooked firm to the bite.
5. Serve warm with the meatballs on top of the noodles. Pour some extra sauce over top of the dish, if desired.

ROSEMARY CHICKEN THIGHS WITH WARM GREENS

Serves 4

Rosemary Chicken Thighs with Warm Greens is a delicious, savory dish that's ready in less than 30 minutes and brimming with greens containing a variety of vitamins and minerals to support adrenal and gut balance. Rosemary adds a lemony flavor and immune-system boost!

1 pound boneless, skinless chicken thighs
2 teaspoons extra-virgin olive oil
Sea salt or pink Himalayan salt to taste
Freshly ground black pepper to taste (if tolerated)
1 tablespoon fresh rosemary, minced
2 tablespoons coconut aminos
1 garlic clove, minced
1 tablespoon coconut oil
2 large leeks, chopped
3 cups kale, chopped
2 cups collard greens, chopped

1. Preheat the oven to 375°F.
2. In a large bowl, toss together the chicken, olive oil, salt, pepper (if tolerated), rosemary, coconut aminos, and garlic.
3. In a large baking dish, pour the contents of the bowl and cover with aluminum foil.
4. Place the baking dish in the oven and bake for 10 minutes.
5. Uncover the baking dish, stir, and cook for 10 minutes more, until the chicken is cooked through.

6. In a large skillet over medium heat, heat the coconut oil. Add the leeks, kale, and collard greens and cover. Cook for 5 minutes, until the greens are tender.
7. Serve the greens warm with the chicken.

SAUSAGE & KALE "PASTA" CASSEROLE
Serves 4

Casseroles are a great way to load up a variety of healing nutrients into one dish! You won't even miss the "real" pasta in this comforting meal. Spaghetti squash adds a nice texture and bite and is a good source of fiber and pantothenic acid, a B vitamin linked to healthy adrenal function.

1 medium spaghetti squash

1 tablespoon coconut oil

Sea salt or pink Himalayan salt to taste

Freshly ground black pepper to taste (if tolerated)

1 pound gluten- and nitrate-free pork sausage

½ cup red onion, sliced

1 garlic clove, minced

2 teaspoons Italian herb seasoning

5 kale leaves, de-stemmed and chopped

⅓ cup bone broth (store-bought, or see recipe on page 305)

½ cup full-fat canned coconut milk

1. Preheat the oven to 400°F.
2. On a large cutting board, cut the squash in half lengthwise. Scoop out the seeds and discard them.
3. Place the halves, cut-side up, on a rimmed baking sheet. Rub with coconut oil and sprinkle with salt and pepper (if tolerated).
4. Roast in the oven for 45 minutes, until you can poke the squash easily with a fork. Let it cool until you can handle it safely. Scrape the insides with a fork to shred the squash into strands.

5. In a large skillet over medium heat, add the sausage and brown it. Once cooked through, set it aside.
6. In the same skillet, add the onion and sauté for 3 minutes. Then add the garlic, Italian seasoning, and kale and cook for 3 minutes more to slightly wilt the kale.
7. Pour in the broth and coconut milk. Simmer for an additional 3 minutes, then remove from the heat.
8. Combine the cooked sausage and the spaghetti squash in the skillet. Stir well.
9. Bake for 15 minutes, uncovered, until the top has slightly browned.

SHRIMP & SQUASH SKEWERS
Serves 4

My Shrimp and Squash Skewers are a barbecue favorite. Marinating the shrimp and vegetables for at least 15 minutes (though no more than 30) pumps up the flavor. Add a squeeze of lemon for a hit of citrus and vitamin C!

1 pound shrimp, shelled and deveined
1 cup zucchini, chopped
1 large bell pepper (any color), sliced thick
1 large red onion, cut into wedges
1 cup mushrooms, halved
2 tablespoons coconut aminos
1 garlic clove, minced
1 tablespoon extra-virgin olive oil
Sea salt or pink Himalayan salt to taste
Freshly ground black pepper to taste (if tolerated)
2 tablespoons avocado oil

1. Heat the grill to medium heat.
2. In a large bowl, toss the shrimp, zucchini, bell pepper, red onions, and

mushrooms together with the coconut aminos, garlic, olive oil, salt, black pepper (if tolerated), and avocado oil. Let marinate for 15 minutes.

3. Thread the shrimp and other vegetables on a skewer, alternating between one piece of shrimp and one piece of vegetable. Discard the remaining marinade.
4. Place the skewers on a preheated grill and cook for 5 minutes (or more) on each side, until the shrimp is opaque and cooked through and the vegetables are tender.
5. Serve warm.

Note

If using wood skewers, soak them in water for 30 minutes prior to threading.

TURKEY & AVOCADO BURRITO
Serves 4

Collard greens are the perfect nutrient-dense and gluten-free way to wrap up this fresh and delicious burrito, filled with B vitamin–rich turkey and avocado, an excellent source of healthy monounsaturated fats and folate.

1 tablespoon extra-virgin olive oil or coconut oil

1 pound ground turkey

1 small onion, diced

½ cup mushrooms, chopped

Sea salt or pink Himalayan salt to taste

Freshly ground black pepper to taste (if tolerated)

1 garlic clove, minced

4 large collard green leaves

3 tablespoons fresh cilantro, chopped

1 large avocado, sliced

1 lime, sliced into wedges

1. In a large skillet over medium heat, add the oil.
2. Add the turkey, onion, mushrooms, salt, pepper (if tolerated), and garlic to the skillet and sauté for 10 minutes, until the turkey is cooked through and the vegetables are tender.
3. Spoon the turkey mixture into the collard leaves, then top with cilantro and avocado.
4. Squeeze a wedge of lime over the meat and avocado.
5. Roll up leaves and serve.

TURKEY BREAKFAST SAUSAGE
Serves 4

Don't let the name fool you. My Turkey Breakfast Sausage makes a simple, satisfying lunch and dinner, too! Try swapping the baby spinach for other leafy greens, like Swiss chard, to change up the flavor profile.

1 pound ground turkey

2 teaspoons ground sage

1 teaspoon fresh rosemary, chopped

1 teaspoon fresh thyme, chopped

½ teaspoon garlic powder

½ teaspoon ground cinnamon

Sea salt or pink Himalayan salt to taste

Freshly ground black pepper to taste (if tolerated)

2 tablespoons coconut oil

4 cups baby spinach

1. In a medium bowl, combine and mix the turkey, sage, rosemary, thyme, garlic powder, cinnamon, salt, and pepper (if tolerated). Refrigerate for at least 30 minutes to firm the meat mixture.
2. Once the mixture has been chilled, form into patties and place on a lined plate.

3. In a large skillet, heat the coconut oil over medium heat. Once the oil is hot, add the patties. Cook for 5 minutes per side, or until no longer pink in the middle.
4. Add the baby spinach and cook until wilted.
5. Serve warm.

HEARTY BEEF STEW

Serves 8

A batch of Hearty Beef Stew usually yields about 8 servings, perfect for leftovers over a couple of days or to store in the freezer for a later date. Bonus: This stew tastes even better the next day, when all of the flavors have had more time to meld!

¼ cup arrowroot flour

Sea salt or pink Himalayan sea salt to taste

2 pounds stewing beef

2 tablespoons coconut oil

2 large carrots, diced

1 large onion, sliced

3 stalks celery, chopped

2 parsnips, peeled and chopped

8 ounces mushrooms, sliced

1 teaspoon dried oregano

1 teaspoon dried parsley

½ teaspoon dried thyme

3 to 4 cups bone broth (store-bought, or see recipe on page 305)

1. Mix the arrowroot flour and salt together in a shallow bowl and dredge each piece of beef so that each piece has a light coating of the flour mixture.
2. Heat the coconut oil over medium heat in a large skillet and brown the beef in batches.

3. Transfer the beef to a slow cooker and add the carrots, onion, celery, parsnips, mushrooms, oregano, parsley, and thyme.
4. Stir the meat and vegetables together until well mixed, then pour the bone broth over the mixture until the liquid just covers the ingredients. (If you have leftover bone broth, heat it up and enjoy a warm mug!)
5. Cook over low heat for 8 hours, or until the desired tenderness is reached.
6. Alternatively, sauté the beef in an electric pressure cooker on the sauté setting, then add the vegetables and broth until the pot is two-thirds full. Turn the pressure cooker to manual and set the pressure on high for 45 minutes.

Note
This stew is great for leftovers and can be frozen for reheating.

CUBAN ROPA VIEJA
Serves 8

While shredded beef is traditionally used to make ropa vieja ("old clothes"), one of Cuba's most popular dishes, I also like to use buffalo chuck steak. Increasingly readily available and affordable, bison is high in protein, iron, zinc, selenium, and B vitamins. Give it a try!

1½ pounds boneless beef or buffalo chuck steak

1 cup sliced onion

½ cup diced tomatoes

1 tablespoon tomato paste

1 tablespoon extra-virgin olive oil

1 tablespoon apple cider vinegar

1 tablespoon garlic, minced

1 teaspoon ground cumin (if tolerated)

1 bay leaf

½ teaspoon sea salt or pink Himalayan sea salt

¼ cup green olives, pitted

⅓ cup fresh cilantro

1 cup bone broth (store-bought, or see recipe on page 305)

1. Place the beef, onion, tomatoes, tomato paste, olive oil, vinegar, garlic, cumin (if tolerated), bay leaf, salt, olives, cilantro, and bone broth in a slow cooker and cook on low for 8 to 10 hours, until the steak is very tender. (Alternatively, place all of the ingredients in an electric pressure cooker and, on manual, set the pressure to high for 50 minutes.)
2. Remove the steak from the slow cooker (or pressure cooker) and shred with two forks. Discard the bay leaf.
3. If there is too much liquid in the pot, turn the slow cooker to high, with the lid off, to reduce the liquid (or use the sauté setting on the electric pressure cooker to reduce the liquid).
4. Serve warm.

BIGOS (POLISH HUNTER'S STEW)
Serves 6

Bigos, also known as Hunter's Stew, is considered a Polish national dish and is often served during the cold winter months, but I encourage you to enjoy this hearty dish whenever you need an extra nutrient boost. In Poland, every family has its own version of this recipe—some include wild meats like rabbit, others include plums—but it always consists of various meats, vegetables, and spices that are stewed with cabbage, one of the key ingredients. Traditionally, Bigos is made on the stovetop, but I make mine in a slow cooker; I love the fact that I can make a big batch and eat it for a few days!

2 (24-ounce) jars of sauerkraut or 1 large cabbage, shredded (about 6 cups)

2 cups shredded vegetables, such as celery, broccoli, and/or carrots (optional)

16 ounces boneless chicken breast, cubed

1 pound ground turkey, beef, or pork

1 tablespoon dried basil

1 tablespoon paprika (if tolerated)

1 teaspoon sea salt or pink Himalayan sea salt

1 bay leaf

1 cup water

1. Place the sauerkraut, vegetables (if using), chicken, turkey, basil, paprika (if tolerated), salt, bay leaf, and water in a slow cooker, mix, and cook on low for 6 to 8 hours. Discard the bay leaf.
2. Serve warm.

CHICKEN TANDOORI

Serves 4 to 6

This delicious slow cooker version of Chicken Tandoori is a weeknight and dinner-party favorite. Curcumin, found in turmeric and curry powder, is gut-healing, liver-supporting, and anti-inflammatory.

1 chicken, cut into pieces, or 8 chicken drumsticks

1 teaspoon turmeric

1 teaspoon paprika (if tolerated)

1 teaspoon curry powder (if tolerated)

1 teaspoon garlic powder

1 teaspoon sea salt or pink Himalayan sea salt

½ teaspoon freshly ground black pepper (if tolerated)

2 cups full-fat canned coconut milk

1. Place the chicken, turmeric, paprika (if tolerated), curry powder (if tolerated), garlic powder, salt, pepper (if tolerated), and coconut milk in a slow cooker and cook on low for 6 to 8 hours, until the chicken is cooked through.
2. Serve warm.

PULLED CHERRY PORK
Serves 8

Antioxidant-rich and inflammation-fighting tart cherries are the perfect complement to tender pork. Serve alongside Roasted Broccoli (page 326) or Cauliflower Mash (page 327) for a flavor-packed meal that's sure to impress.

3 to 4 pounds boneless pork ribs or chicken (dark meat)

1 cup frozen tart cherries, pitted

6 garlic cloves

½ cup coconut aminos

½ cup apple cider vinegar

1 cup cherry juice

⅓ cup maple syrup

1. Place the meat, cherries, and garlic in a slow cooker.
2. In a large bowl, combine the coconut aminos, vinegar, cherry juice, and maple syrup and pour this mixture over the meat.
3. Cover and cook on high for 5 to 6 hours, or on low for 10 to 12 hours, until the meat is cooked through and tender.
4. Serve warm.

HEARTY CHICKEN SOUP
Serves 8

My Hearty Chicken Soup is like a hug from the inside! Brimming with vegetables and cubed chicken, this soup satisfies, even without noodles. If you'd like noodles, however, add some zucchini noodles for extra fiber and nutrients.

2 tablespoons coconut oil

1 large onion, chopped

1 bay leaf

2 garlic cloves

Sea salt or pink Himalayan salt to taste

Freshly ground black pepper to taste (if tolerated)

8 cups bone broth (store-bought, or see recipe on page 305)

1 pound chicken

3 large turnips, chopped

1 large celeriac, chopped

4 large carrots, chopped

1. In a large pot over medium-high heat, heat the coconut oil and add the onion, bay leaf, garlic, salt, and pepper (if tolerated). Cook for 5 to 7 minutes, until the onions start to brown.
2. Transfer to a slow cooker and add the bone broth, chicken, turnips, celeriac, and carrots to the pot.
3. Set the temperature to low and slow cook for 6 to 8 hours.
4. Remove the chicken meat from the bones and add the meat back to the soup. Discard the bones and the bay leaf.
5. Season to taste as needed with salt and pepper and serve warm.

ASIAN SESAME ROAST BEEF

Serves 8

With a little effort, Asian Sesame Roast Beef delivers a super-flavorful and tender dish that's better than any takeout. Immune-supporting sesame seeds add crunch, while warm, spicy ginger provides digestive support.

1 beef roast (about 3 pounds)

1 tablespoon fresh ginger, minced

Sea salt or pink Himalayan salt to taste

Freshly ground black pepper to taste (if tolerated)

2 teaspoons sesame seeds

2 tablespoons freshly squeezed lime juice

2 tablespoons lime zest

1 teaspoon sesame oil

¾ cup bone broth (store-bought, or see recipe on page 305)

2 cups carrots, steamed

2 cups bok choy, steamed

1. Place the beef roast in a large zipper-top bag.
2. In a small bowl, combine the ginger, salt, pepper (if tolerated), sesame seeds, lime juice, lime zest, sesame oil, and bone broth and mix well to create a sauce.
3. Pour the sauce into the bag and seal it, squeezing out any excess air. Turn the bag over to coat the roast evenly.
4. Refrigerate the bag for 2 hours.
5. Empty the contents of the bag into a large slow cooker. Add the carrots and bok choy.
6. Cover and cook on low for 6 to 9 hours, until the beef is very tender.
7. Using two forks, shred the beef into bite-sized pieces and serve with vegetables.

SLOW-COOKED CHICKEN WITH ROASTED PARSNIPS
Serves 8

Nothing says family dinner like a slow-cooked chicken seasoned with fragrant herbs cooked to golden perfection. High in vitamin C, roasted parsnips bring immune-system support without the blood sugar swing associated with the traditional side of white potatoes.

1 whole chicken, insides removed

3 tablespoons coconut oil

Sea salt or pink Himalayan salt to taste

Freshly ground black pepper to taste (if tolerated)

2 tablespoons fresh sage, chopped

2 tablespoons fresh rosemary, chopped

1 lemon, quartered

3 cups fresh parsnips, chopped

1. Place the chicken on a large cutting board.
2. Use your fingers to loosen the skin away from the chicken meat.
3. In a small bowl, combine 2 tablespoons of the coconut oil with the salt, pepper (if tolerated), sage, and rosemary and form a paste.
4. Rub the paste under the skin of the chicken.
5. Squeeze the lemon quarters into the cavity and place the squeezed lemon inside.
6. Place the chicken in a large slow cooker, then cover and cook on low for 6 hours, or until the chicken is falling off the bone and cooked through.
7. Let cool slightly and remove the chicken from the bones. Set it aside and keep warm.
8. Preheat the oven to 375°F.
9. Line a large baking sheet with parchment paper and set aside.
10. In a large bowl, toss the parsnips with the remaining tablespoon of coconut oil. Season the parsnip mixture with salt and pepper (if tolerated).
11. On the prepared baking sheet, place the parsnip mixture and spread it out evenly.
12. Bake the mixture for 20 minutes, flipping halfway, until the parsnips are tender and crisp.
13. Serve warm alongside the chicken meat.

SLOW-COOKED LONDON BROIL WITH TURNIP & ARUGULA SALAD

Serves 6 to 8

Tender, iron-rich beef pairs nicely with the peppery kick of arugula in this full-flavored salad.

1 (1½- to 2-pound) London broil

1 tablespoon extra-virgin olive oil

¼ cup coconut aminos

1 garlic clove, minced

1 tablespoon fresh ginger, grated

Sea salt or pink Himalayan salt to taste

Freshly ground black pepper to taste (if tolerated)

¼ cup bone broth (store-bought, or see recipe on page 305)

1 cup turnips, chopped

1 cup arugula, chopped

¼ cup freshly squeezed lime juice

2 tablespoons fresh basil, chopped

2 garlic cloves, peeled and minced

1. Place the meat in a large resealable bag.
2. In a medium bowl, whisk together the olive oil, coconut aminos, garlic, ginger, salt, and pepper (if tolerated) to make the marinade.
3. Pour the marinade over the meat and seal the bag.
4. Refrigerate the bag for at least 2 hours.
5. Add the London broil and the bone broth to a large slow cooker.
6. Cover and cook on low for 6 to 8 hours, until the meat is very tender.
7. Add the turnips in the last hour.
8. Allow the meat to cool, then slice.
9. In a medium bowl, toss the beef and turnips with the arugula.
10. In a small bowl, whisk together the lime juice, basil, and garlic to make the dressing, and add salt and pepper (if tolerated) to taste.
11. Pour the dressing over the salad, then toss and serve.

Sides

APPLE CINNAMON CABBAGE SAUTÉ
Serves 4

Sautés are a quick, simple side for any meal, and cabbage is a wonderfully versatile base—and detoxifying crucifer! Here, it's combined with warming, blood sugar–balancing cinnamon and fiber-rich apples.

1 tablespoon coconut oil

1 small cabbage (any variety), cored and sliced thin

2 carrots, peeled and grated

2 large onions, peeled and sliced thin

1 apple, cored and sliced into matchstick-size pieces

1 teaspoon ground turmeric

1 teaspoon ground cinnamon

½ teaspoon ground ginger

Sea salt to taste

Freshly ground black pepper to taste (if tolerated)

Freshly squeezed juice of ½ organic lemon

1. In a large skillet, heat the coconut oil over medium heat.
2. Add the cabbage, carrots, and onions. Cook for 15 minutes, or until wilted.
3. Add the apple, turmeric, cinnamon, ginger, salt, and pepper (if tolerated) and sauté for another 5 to 7 minutes, until the apple is softened.
4. Add the lemon juice and stir to combine.
5. Serve warm or cold.

ROASTED BROCCOLI

Serves 4

Broccoli is a nutritional powerhouse, loaded with fiber, vitamin C, and folate, and it's one of my favorite ways to amp up the vitamins and minerals in any meal. Roasting enhances the flavor and creates deliciously crispy tips!

1 head of broccoli, cored and separated

2 tablespoons extra-virgin olive oil

Sea salt or pink Himalayan salt to taste

Freshly ground black pepper to taste (if tolerated)

Freshly squeezed juice of 1 organic lemon

1. Preheat the oven to 350°F.
2. Line a rimmed baking sheet with parchment paper (you may need to use two baking sheets).
3. Add the broccoli to the middle of the baking sheet(s) and drizzle the olive oil over top.
4. Sprinkle it with salt and pepper (if tolerated) and mix everything with your hands.
5. Spread the broccoli evenly over the baking sheet(s).
6. Bake for 20 minutes, or until the edges of the broccoli turn brown.
7. Remove from the oven and sprinkle with lemon juice.

CAULIFLOWER MASH
Serves 4

If you're looking for a healthier alternative to mashed potatoes, look no further than this creamy Cauliflower Mash! Coconut milk adds healthy fats and a rich, velvety texture, while cauliflower is an excellent detoxifying source of fiber, vitamin C, and B vitamins, and its mild flavor pairs well with any spice or herb.

1 head of cauliflower

⅓ cup full-fat canned coconut milk

Sea salt or pink Himalayan salt (or truffle sea salt if you have a Trader Joe's nearby)

¼ cup fresh chives, parsley, or dill, minced, plus more for sprinkling on top

1. Steam the cauliflower until very tender.
2. Break up the cauliflower into smaller pieces and add to the bowl of a high-speed blender, like the Vitamix, or place the cauliflower in a bowl and mash with a potato masher.
3. Stir in the coconut milk, salt, and herbs.
4. Top with fresh herbs.

CUCUMBER & TOMATO SALAD

Serves 4

Light and refreshing, Cucumber and Tomato Salad has a regular place on my summertime picnic table, when tomatoes are at their most flavorful.

1 large cucumber, sliced and quartered

2 cups cherry tomatoes, sliced (quartered if they are large)

¼ cup extra-virgin olive oil

⅛ cup apple cider vinegar

Sea salt or pink Himalayan salt to taste

Freshly ground black pepper to taste (if tolerated)

1 tablespoon mixed dried herbs of choice (like parsley, oregano, and rosemary)

1. Place the cucumber and tomatoes in a medium bowl.
2. Whisk together the olive oil, vinegar, salt, pepper (if tolerated), and herbs until combined to make the dressing.
3. Pour the dressing over the vegetables and serve.

ROASTED ROOT VEGETABLES

Serves 8

With an endless combination of vegetables and herbs, this classic side dish never gets boring. Roasting is a simple, no-fuss way to prepare a big batch of veggies—perfect for leftovers throughout the week.

1 bunch radishes, trimmed and chopped

4 small sweet potatoes, scrubbed and chopped

4 medium beets, peeled and chopped

1 small butternut squash, peeled, seeded, and chopped

1 head of broccoli, chopped

½ pound Brussels sprouts, halved

2 tablespoons coconut oil or avocado oil, melted

1 tablespoon dried herbs of choice

Sea salt or pink Himalayan salt to taste

Freshly ground black pepper to taste (if tolerated)

1. Preheat the oven to 400°F.
2. In a large bowl, combine the radishes, sweet potatoes, beets, butternut squash, broccoli, and Brussels sprouts with the melted coconut oil and mix well.
3. Add the herbs, salt, and pepper (if tolerated) and mix again, until evenly distributed.
4. On a rimmed baking sheet (you may need two), spread the vegetables evenly and bake until cooked through. (Note: This may take 1 to 2 hours, depending on how soft you like your vegetables.)

Note

You can add or remove vegetables to create your own combinations.

SAUTÉED SPINACH

Serves 2

Sautéed Spinach is a nutritious, delicious side that's ready in a snap. Be careful not to overcook the spinach, and don't skip the lemon juice for a splash of vitamin C and detox support!

1 tablespoon extra-virgin olive oil

2 garlic cloves, minced

10 ounces baby spinach

Sea salt or pink Himalayan salt to taste

Freshly ground black pepper to taste (if tolerated)

Freshly squeezed juice of ½ lemon

1. In a large pan over medium heat, add the olive oil.
2. Add the garlic and sauté for 1 minute.
3. Add the spinach and stir for 2 minutes, or until wilted.

4. Sprinkle the spinach with salt, pepper (if tolerated), and lemon juice and serve warm.

Snacks

BACON, MUSHROOM & EGG MUFFINS
Serves 6

Eggs aren't only for breakfast! Protein-rich eggs and bacon and selenium-packed mushrooms make for a satisfying snack at any time of day and are easy to take on the go.

½ pound bacon, chopped

1½ cups mushrooms, chopped

2 tablespoons green onion, chopped

½ teaspoon fresh thyme, chopped

6 large eggs, beaten

Sea salt or pink Himalayan salt to taste

Freshly ground black pepper to taste (if tolerated)

1. Preheat the oven to 350°F.
2. In a large skillet over medium heat, add the bacon, mushrooms, green onion, and thyme.
3. Cook for 5 to 10 minutes, until the bacon is crispy and the vegetables are tender.
4. Place a spoonful of the bacon mixture into each section of a paper-lined muffin tin (you should have enough to evenly fill 10 to 12 rounds).
5. Evenly pour the beaten eggs over each section. Season with salt and pepper (if tolerated).
6. Place in the oven and bake for 10 minutes, until the eggs are firm.
7. Serve warm.

CHIA PUDDING

Serves 4

Loaded with protein, fiber, and healthy fats, Chia Pudding is a creamy and simple-to-make snack.

1 cup full-fat canned coconut milk
2 tablespoons chia seeds
½ cup strawberries and raspberries (or other desired fruit), chopped
Stevia to taste (optional)

1. Mix the coconut milk, chia seeds, strawberries and raspberries, and stevia (if using) in a small Mason jar or in 4 ramekins.
2. Chill for 4 hours, until firm.

DELI WRAPS/BELL PEPPER SANDWICH

Serves 1

Sometimes you just want a sandwich! Collard greens and red peppers make for nutritious, gluten-free "bread" with a satisfying crunch.

1 large collard green leaf or 1 large bell pepper
Assorted nitrate- and additive-free deli meats or fresh-cooked chicken, turkey,
    or beef, sliced
Greens of choice, such as microgreens
Condiments of choice, such as mustard or guacamole

Collard Wraps
1. Fill a large collard green leaf with meat, greens, and condiments.
2. Roll everything up like a wrap.

Bell Pepper Sandwich

1. Slice one whole bell pepper in half, then core.
2. Fill one side of the pepper with meat, greens, and condiments.
3. Place the other half of the bell pepper on top and squish down to make it flat. (Don't worry if the pepper cracks a little!)

DEVILED EGGS—ADRENAL STYLE

Serves 6

If you love thick, creamy mayonnaise, you'll love the Paleo-compliant version made with fats like avocado oil instead of vegetable oil. There are many store-bought or homemade options available to add richness and flavor to these Deviled Eggs. Sprinkle with turmeric for a pop of color and gut-healing boost!

3 large eggs, hard-boiled, peeled, and halved
1 tablespoon Paleo-compliant mayonnaise
½ teaspoon ground turmeric
Sea salt or pink Himalayan salt to taste
Freshly ground black pepper to taste (if tolerated)
Chopped chives, for garnish

1. In a small bowl, scoop out the yolks from the hard-boiled eggs. Set aside the egg white cups.
2. Add the mayonnaise, turmeric, salt, and pepper (if tolerated) to the yolks. Mix the yolk mixture with a spoon until smooth.
3. Scoop the yolk mixture into the egg white cups and top with chives.
4. Serve cold.

GUACAMOLE & CRUDITÉS

Serves 4

Rich in good fats, this soft and crunchy dish makes an excellent snack to keep blood sugar levels stable.

½ cup avocado, diced

⅛ cup red onion, diced

2 tablespoons freshly squeezed lime juice

2 tablespoons extra-virgin olive oil

Various vegetables (such as carrots, cucumber, celery stalks, and bell peppers)

1. In a large bowl, combine the avocado, onion, lime juice, and olive oil. Mash to make guacamole.
2. Cut the vegetables and serve alongside the guacamole.

LIVER PÂTÉ

Serves 8

Liver is one of the richest sources of adrenal-supporting iron and vitamin A, but it is not most people's favorite. Even if you haven't liked liver in the past, I hope you'll try this Liver Pâté recipe I make at home—it's full of other bold flavors that help balance out the richness of the liver.

1 pound beef, chicken, or pork liver, cut into chunks

1 onion, chopped

1 tablespoon duck fat or coconut oil

1 tablespoon coconut fat from coconut milk

1 garlic clove, crushed

¼ cup fresh basil, chopped

4 teaspoons apple cider vinegar

Freshly squeezed juice of ½ lemon

1 tablespoon ground cinnamon

Sea salt or pink Himalayan sea salt to taste

Freshly ground black pepper to taste (if tolerated)

Pickles, for garnish

1. Fry the liver and onion in a pan with the duck fat until cooked through. This should take 5 to 7 minutes.
2. Place the liver and onion along with the coconut fat, garlic, basil, vinegar, lemon juice, cinnamon, salt, and pepper in the bowl of a food processor and blend until smooth.
3. Form the mixture into a ball and chill for an hour.
4. Slice the mixture into thick slices and garnish with pickles.

Gratitude/Acknowledgments

I have found healing comes from community, and I am so grateful to the beautiful people in my own life who supported me over the last few years!

My husband, Michael—I'm so lucky to have you as my soul mate and love you and do life with you. Thank you for always believing in me and thank you for all of the "adventuring" you did with Dimitry before my book deadlines.

My son, Dimitry—for being my greatest teacher and for bringing so much snuggling, fun, joy, love, and laughter into our lives!

My parents, Marta and Adam, who have been there for me my entire life—you are the definition of supportive parents, and I hope to be the same for my Dimitry! I can't thank you enough!

My brother and sister in love, Robert and Amanda Nowosadzki—thank you for your grounding presence in my life! I love you both!

Julia Pastore—thank you for working your magic in turning the Adrenal Transformation Program into a truly transformational and approachable book. I appreciate your brilliant mind, your guidance, your patience, your attention to detail, and the amount of love and care you put into making this book a reality. One book done, seventeen more to go. ☺

I am fortunate to personally know the best healers in the world, and many of them have helped me become the healer that I am today.

Carter Black, RPh, thank you for showing a skeptical pharmacist that treatments for adrenal fatigue can help, and for putting me on a journey to support my adrenals. I also appreciate all of our collaborations!

The trailblazers of adrenal health who shared their knowledge before me, including my mentor Dan Kalish and the late William G. Timmins, James L. Wilson, Marcelle Pick, Thomas Guillams, Alan Christianson, and Carrie Jones. Thank you for passing on your knowledge and teaching others.

My mentors and business coaches, JJ Virgin and Karl Krummenacher—thank you for showing me how to create a business that allows me to help people while keeping myself healthy!

My fellow health and wellness friends and experts, Steve Wright, Magdalena Wszelaki, Debbie and Roy Steinbock, Sheila Kilbane, Christine Maren, Pejman Katerai, Jill Carnahan, David Tusek, Elena Koles, Nicole Beurkens, Christa Orecchio, Katie Wells, James Maskell, Dave Asprey, Trudy Scott, Jolene Brighten, Amy Medling, Brian Mowll, Robyn Openshaw, Elisa Song, Ben Lynch, Mariza Snyder, Ritamarie Loscalzo, Ari Whitten, Courtney Hunt, Oscar Sellerach, and Donna Gates. Some of you helped with providing health consultations for me and my family during scary and uncertain times, some of you served as mentors and friends, and others may have had a conversation with me or even posted something on social media that meant the world to me! Your wisdom helped me go from surviving to thriving during the delicate time of my matrescence and helped me solidify my thoughts on Adrenal Transformation. Please keep shining your light and know that you are making a difference!

My wonderful team:

Brittany—thank you for helping me organize the healing protocol puzzles in my head into real-world actionable solutions, and thank you for tackling each project big or small with such grace, courage, and determination!

Stephanie—thank you for providing your expertise in creating the program recipes and meal plans while meeting some crazy deadlines—all with a smile on your face!

Tina—thank you for sharing your multidimensional talents, from project managing like a ninja to your artistic gifts (and puns), with the world!

Christine, Robin, Katie, and Mindy—thank you for making sure our content is accessible to the people that need it most through your work on customer service, social media, and the website!

Tiziana—thank you for taking care of our ATP participants with so much love and care.

Renee—thank you for jumping in with edits, your great suggestions for flow, and for your flexibility.

Sarah, Diane, and Christin—I appreciate your wordsmithery, research, and inspiring copywriting.

Dave—thank you for creating images to make our content more engaging and memorable!

My literary agents, Celeste Fine and John Maas, and the rest of the fabulous team at Park & Fine. Thank you for your constant support and guidance.

The entire talented team at Avery, especially Lucia Watson and Suzy Swartz. Thank you for getting *Adrenal Transformation Protocol* out into the world!

Dimitry's fun and caring nanny, Deanna ("Durda"), who inspired me to get back into art therapy and allowed me to have the time to create the ATP back in Colorado, as well as his wonderful preschool teachers, who allowed me to come out of "semi-retirement" and taught him Spanish and Mandarin while I worked on this manuscript. Thank you for sharing your teaching and for caring for my little one, so I can share my teaching and care with the world!

My clients and my readers—thank you for trusting me with your health! I'm so proud to be a part of your healing journeys and still get tears in my eyes with every success story! Remember that you can get better!

Advanced Stress Symptom Formulary

ADRENAL DYSFUNCTION TESTING

While the protocols in this program will benefit every stage and pattern of adrenal dysfunction, if you are still struggling with symptoms, or did not tolerate or utilize parts of the protocol, further testing may help with determining other potential interventions more specific to your individualized hormone levels and patterns.

The DUTCH (Dried Urine Test for Comprehensive Hormones) Test

This test assesses your adrenal function through urine testing. I like this test because it measures four or five samples throughout the day to measure cortisol levels, providing a good sense of the daily cortisol rhythm. Another benefit is that you don't have to stop any supplements or protocols in order to do the test.

Adrenal Stress Profile Test by ZRT Laboratory

This test measures four cortisol readings throughout the day, cortisol sum, and DHEA. You may need to stop caffeine and some supplements to ensure accurate testing.

Further Interventions That Support Adrenal Dysfunction Stages

Please consult a knowledgeable practitioner before considering these supplements, as some of them may not be appropriate for you, and appropriate dosing and monitoring are critical.

Pregnenolone

Known as the "mother hormone," pregnenolone is the precursor to all other hormones produced by the adrenals and can help support cortisol levels. Contraindications: history of hormone-dependent cancers or tumors, hyperthyroidism. Brand: BioMatrix Pregnenolone (sublingual drops).

Progesterone

A critical female sex hormone that helps the body prepare and maintain pregnancy, metabolize fat, and maintain stable moods. It has a calming effect on the brain and promotes sleep. Bioidentical, or natural, progesterone may benefit those with low progesterone. You will want to test hormone levels and consult with a practitioner for proper dosing. Designs for Health Progest-Avail Topical Serum contains a super-micronized form of progesterone in triglyceride that facilitates better absorption than conventional creams or compounded topical progesterone (prescription required).

DHEA or 7-Keto

Touted as the "youth hormone," DHEA is the precursor to the hormones estrogen and testosterone. Contraindications: hormone-dependent cancers, tumors, estrogen dominance, high DHEA, high testosterone, or hyperthyroidism. Excess dosing and conversion to other androgens may cause acne; in that case, reduce dose or discontinue. Brand: BioMatrix DHEA (sublingual drops).

Hydrocortisone

This prescription medication can be used when we need more cortisol, as hydrocortisone turns into cortisol within the body. Hydrocortisone may be helpful in the late phase of Stage III adrenal dysfunction when one's total cortisol sum is under 15 nmol/L (flatlined cortisol). Numerous precautions and side effects, including adrenal/pituitary suppression.

Adrenal and pituitary glandulars

In some cases, glandular extracts of the adrenals and pituitary may be utilized to provide further support and balance. Whole-gland extracts may contain adrenaline. Risk of adrenal/pituitary suppression. Some brands of quality glandulars include Standard Process, Biotics Research, and Allergy Research Group.

Licorice root drops (not deglycyrrhizinated licorice, or DGL)

These can help boost low cortisol readings by extending the life of cortisol. Contraindications: high blood pressure. Brand: BioMatrix Licorice Root Extract.

Phosphatidylserine

This promotes the clearance of cortisol from the body and may be utilized for overactive adrenals that produce too much cortisol. Contraindications: Stage III adrenal fatigue.

BLOOD SUGAR SUPPORT

Related Stress Symptoms

- Brain fog and fatigue (BFF)
- Insomnia and sleep issues (ISI)
- Libido (L)
- Mood (M)
- Pain (P)

Supplement Support

Myo-inositol has been used in doses as high as 18 grams per day for obsessive-compulsive disorder. A starting dose may be 3 grams per day in three divided doses.

Adding additional amino acids can help with balancing blood sugar and the related anxiety in some. Amino-NR (Pure Encapsulations) to be taken three times per day. Others have also benefited from using l-Glutamine (Pure Encapsulations) for low blood sugar (starting with 500 mg per day).

Berberine and chromium have also been found to help stabilize blood sugar. See Blood Sugar Support Supplements (page 343) for more.

Test for Reactive Hypoglycemia

You can easily test yourself for reactive hypoglycemia with the use of an over-the-counter blood glucose monitoring kit, which uses a small finger prick to collect a sample of your blood. Follow these instructions to test your reactions:

- After at least ten hours of fasting (such as first thing in the morning), test your blood sugar before eating your first meal of the day.
- Eat a meal with your typical carbohydrate serving.
- Record the meal in a journal.
- Repeat testing every thirty minutes, for a total of four hours.
- Repeat as necessary to test other foods.

A surprising thing I've learned over the years is that different foods may produce different reactions. I suspect this is largely connected to our unique mix of genetics, health conditions, digestive enzymes, and nutrients that determine how we "process" each unique food molecule.

If blood sugar levels drop below 70 mg/dL at any time during this four-hour period, this could be an indication that you are experiencing reactive hypoglycemia. If so, consult with your doctor to discuss treatment options.

For more detailed real-time readings, your doctor may prescribe a continuous glucose monitor, which uses a sensor placed under your skin or adhered to the back of your arm to automatically collect your blood sugar levels every five to fifteen minutes. The readings are sent to a monitor that both you and your doctor can review to help identify what could be causing the fluctuations and make more informed decisions about how to resolve them. This has been a game-changer for many individuals who have had trouble stabilizing their blood sugar with other interventions.

Blood Sugar Support Supplements

Supplement	Symptoms	Recommended Product, Dose, and Notes
Amino acids	M	Pure Encapsulations Amino-NR, three times per day
Berberine	ISI, M	Rootcology Berberine, Designs for Health Berb-Evail, follow package
Chromium	ISI, M	Pure Encapsulations ChromeMate GTF, 600 mcg per day
L-Glutamine	M	Pure Encapsulations l-Glutamine, start with 500 mg per day

ENZYMES
Related Stress Symptoms
- Brain fog and fatigue (BFF)
- Pain (P)

A lack of enzymes can make it difficult to digest various foods and products of metabolism and cellular function, which can set off a chain reaction of digestive trouble, including leaky gut, food sensitivities, nutrient depletions, and widespread inflammation associated with multiple adrenal symptoms, such as brain fog, fatigue, insomnia, and sleep issues.

Discovering that I had a deficiency of stomach acid was a huge aha moment for me. After I started taking betaine with pepsin, my ten-year-long debilitating fatigue was lifted practically overnight, and I went from sleeping for eleven to twelve hours per night to eight hours. I immediately began feeling more rested and energetic—just because I started digesting my food better. The following six types of enzymes may be especially beneficial in supporting good digestion:

Broad-Spectrum Enzymes

For Inflammation and Pain Reduction: Systemic Enzymes

Systemic enzymes, also known as proteolytic enzymes, speed up tissue repair, act as natural immune modulators, and help break down gut pathogens and self-tissue antibodies that are present in autoimmune conditions and lead to inflammation.

They are not to be taken with food but rather on an empty stomach, at least forty-five minutes before a meal, or one and a half hours after a meal. Otherwise, they will get used up in the process of digestion instead of getting into the bloodstream to act on circulating immune complexes.

Most labels of systemic enzymes recommend six capsules daily with a glass of water (at least 8 ounces).

If no response is experienced, clinicians may sometimes use five to ten capsules, three times per day, in the acute phase to modulate the immune system effectively. I recommend talking with your practitioner about higher doses, if you don't see results with the starting dose.

Broad-Spectrum Digestive Enzymes

Broad-spectrum digestive enzymes contain a variety of ingredients that promote the breakdown of a wide range of nutrients, including fiber, starch, fat, and protein.

They may contain enzymes derived from plants, animals, or herbs to promote natural digestive enzyme activity and bile flow.

Herbal formulations may offer the advantage of providing gentle but broad digestive support and may be a great option for those who find hydrochloric acid irritating or cannot take animal-derived enzymes.

Enzymes for Specific Types of Foods

For Protein Digestion: Betaine with Pepsin

Low stomach acid makes it more difficult to digest protein, contributing to a host of symptoms, including brain fog, depression, fatigue, insomnia and sleep issues, and pain, among others, as well as the development of food sensitivities and an imbalanced gut microbiome.

Low stomach acid can result from adrenal issues that deplete our chloride stores (a vicious cycle!), nutrient deficiencies (such as thiamine), a vegetarian or vegan diet, and infections like *H. pylori* that neutralize stomach acid to aid their survival.

To support low stomach acid and promote good digestion and nutrient absorption, I recommend supplementing with betaine and pepsin. Betaine HCl (also known as betaine hydrochloride) and pepsin are naturally occurring components of gastric juice that break down protein to make nutrients and amino acids from our protein-containing foods more bioavailable.

Betaine with pepsin should be taken with a protein-rich meal, starting with one capsule per meal.

The dose should be increased by one more capsule at each meal, until symptoms of too much acid are felt (burping, burning, warming in the stomach region, etc.). At that point, you will know that your dose is one capsule less than what resulted in symptoms.

Drinking a mixture of one teaspoon of baking soda in a glass of water can reduce these temporary symptoms.

Dosing example:

Meal No. 1: Took one capsule, didn't feel symptoms

Meal No. 2: Took two capsules, didn't feel symptoms

Meal No. 3: Took three capsules, didn't feel symptoms

Meal No. 4: Took four capsules, felt symptoms

Target dose: Three capsules

For Fat Digestion: Pancreatic Enzymes and/or
Bile-Supporting Enzymes

Some signs and symptoms of poor fat digestion/fat malabsorption include frequent diarrhea, gas and bloating after eating, stomach pain, cramping, foul-smelling and greasy stools, and weight loss, as well as a low fecal elastase on a stool test.

- You may also experience symptoms related to essential fatty-acid deficiency as well as depletions in the fat-soluble vitamins (A, D, E, and K).
- A deficiency in pancreatic enzymes (amylase, lipase, and protease) or bile can lead to fat malabsorption.

- Pancreatic enzymes and/or enzymes with ox bile and/or focused on supporting gallbladder function may be used.
- For fat digestive support, the following enzymes can be helpful: Rootcology Liver & Gallbladder Support, Pure Encapsulations Digestion GB, or Designs for Health LV-GB Complex.
- For pancreatic enzyme support in mild cases of insufficiency, a low dose of pancreatic enzymes plus ox bile may be helpful.
  - Rootcology Pancreatic Enzymes Plus can be helpful, as well as Designs for Health PaleoZyme.
- When advanced pancreatic insufficiency is present, higher-dose supplements may be needed, such as Pure Encapsulations Pancreatic Enzymes Formula or the prescription medication Creon.
- In those with gallbladder issues or who have had their gallbladder removed, a bile-supporting blend with ox bile may be indicated.
  - Rootcology Liver & Gallbladder Support
  - Designs for Health LV-GB Complex
  - Pure Encapsulations Digestion GB

For Fiber Digestion: Veggie Enzymes
Symptoms of impaired fiber digestion: bloating and abdominal discomfort after consuming vegetables and fruits, undigested plant fibers in stool.

- May help reduce gas and bloating after meals (especially meals with lots of raw vegetables), constipation, and a feeling of fullness after eating only a small quantity of food, as well as symptoms of nutrient deficiencies that may occur when the body is unable to break down and absorb the nutrients in fibrous vegetables, including fatigue, hair loss, muscle pain, and autoimmunity itself.

Gluten/Dairy Digestive Enzymes: Gluten/Dairy-Targeted Proteases +/- Lactase
A blend of digestive enzymes that help break down gluten, the main reactive protein found in wheat, and casein, the main reactive protein found in dairy. It can minimize reactions when small amounts are accidentally consumed.

- Lactase can prevent reactions from lactose found in dairy products, in those who have lactose intolerance.

Enzyme	How to Use	Recommended Supplement
Systemic Enzymes (proteolytic enzymes), natural immune modulators	Take on an empty stomach, at least forty-five minutes before a meal or one and a half hours after a meal.	Rootcology Systemic Enzymes, Douglas Laboratories Wobenzym N and Wobenzym PS, Pure Encapsulations Systemic Enzyme Complex, Designs for Health Inflammatone
Broad-Spectrum Digestive Enzymes, support the digestion of fiber, starch, and fat.	Take with all meals.	Rootcology Herbal Bitters, Pure Encapsulations Digestive Enzymes Ultra, Designs for Health CarminaGest
Betaine with Pepsin, protein digestive enzymes	Take with protein-rich meals.	Rootcology Betaine with Pepsin, Pure Encapsulations Betaine HCl Pepsin, Designs for Health Betaine HCl
Pancreatic Enzymes, support fat digestion and the healthy absorption of nutrients.	Take with fat-containing meals. In advanced stages of exocrine pancreatic insufficiency, one may require high doses and may need to take multiple pills with each meal and snack, based on one's weight.	Rootcology Pancreatic Enzymes Plus, Designs for Health PaleoZyme (for mild issues)—contain pancreatic enzymes and ox bile Pure Encapsulations Pancreatic Enzymes Formula (for more advanced stages) or Creon (Rx)—contain only pancreatic enzymes
Gallbladder Support with Ox Bile	Take with fat-containing meals.	Rootcology Liver & Gallbladder Support, Pure Encapsulations Digestion GB, Designs for Health LV-GB Complex
Veggie Enzymes, support the digestion of fruits and vegetables.	Take with vegetable- and fiber-rich meals.	Rootcology Veggie Enzymes, Designs for Health Plant Enzyme Digestive Formula
Gluten/Dairy Digestive Enzymes, help minimize reactions to small amounts of gluten and dairy.	Take when eating gluten and/or dairy or accidentally exposed.	Pure Encapsulations Gluten/Dairy Digest, Designs for Health AllerGzyme

HORMONES

Female Hormone Imbalance
Related Stress Symptoms:
- Brain fog and fatigue (BFF)
- Insomnia and sleep issues (ISI)
- Libido (L)
- Mood (M)

Estrogen, the primary female sex hormone, regulates sexual development, reproductive health, and the menstrual cycle while playing essential roles in the optimal functioning of nearly every organ in the body, including the brain. Estrogen also helps regulate several feel-good neurotransmitters such as serotonin and dopamine.

Progesterone, another critical female sex hormone, helps the body prepare and maintain pregnancy, metabolize fat, and maintain stable moods. It has a calming effect on the brain and promotes sleep. These two hormones work best when they are in sync, working together like dance partners to maintain balance.

One of the most common types of imbalance occurs when there is not enough progesterone to balance out estrogen. When this happens, the body can enter a highly inflammatory state known as estrogen dominance, linked to symptoms such as:

- Anxiety, irritability, and mood swings
- Fibroids
- Hot flashes
- Breast lumps and fibrocystic breasts
- Heavy periods or postmenopausal bleeding
- Irregular, sporadic, or absent periods
- Worsening symptoms of PMS (premenstrual syndrome) or PMDD (premenstrual dysphoric disorder)

Many factors contribute to estrogen dominance, including stress, impaired liver function, and an unhealthy gut, but women are especially vulnerable during perimenopause (the transitional period before menopause and the complete absence of menstrual bleeding for at least one year) and menopause, when progesterone levels naturally decline.

If you have had your hormone levels tested and know that you have low progesterone (see Testing), supplementing with topical bioidentical, or natural, progesterone, a cream, gel, or oil rubbed into the skin, can help ease symptoms of estrogen dominance and promote a calmer, more relaxed mindset and better sleep.

Supplement	Symptoms	Recommended Product, Dose, and Notes
Progesterone	BFF, ISI, L, M	Designs for Health Progest-Avail Topical Serum compounded topical progesterone (Rx), work with a practitioner for proper dosing

Please refer to *Cooking for Hormone Balance* and *Overcoming Estrogen Dominance* by Magdalena Wszelaki for more guidance.

Thyroid Hormones
Related Stress Symptoms:
- Brain fog and fatigue (BFF)
- Insomnia and sleep issues (ISI)
- Libido (L)
- Mood (M)
- Pain (P)

Having an imbalance of thyroid hormones can lead to a whole host of issues, including brain fog, fatigue, insomnia and sleep issues, low libido, mood imbalances, and pain. The two most common thyroid conditions are:

- Graves' disease, when the thyroid makes too much thyroid hormone (most common cause of hyperthyroidism)
- Hashimoto's, when the thyroid makes too little hormone (most common cause of hypothyroidism)

Common Symptoms of Hypothyroidism	Common Symptoms of Hyperthyroidism
Cold intolerance	Anxiety
Constipation	Eye protrusion
Depression	Fatigue
Dry skin	Hair loss
Fatigue	Heart palpitations
Forgetfulness	Heat intolerance
Hair loss	Increased appetite
Joint pain	Irritability
Loss of ambition	Menstrual disturbances
Low libido	Muscle loss and pain
Menstrual irregularities	Sleep disturbances
Muscle cramps	Tremors
Stiffness	Weight loss

While symptoms of hyperthyroidism (like anxiety, irritability, insomnia, and palpitations) are commonly attributed to Graves' disease, it's important to note that they can also occur when someone is overmedicated with thyroid hormones and in the early stages of Hashimoto's.

In the early stages of Hashimoto's, when the thyroid is under attack by the immune system, thyroid cells are broken down and release thyroid hormones into the bloodstream. This causes thyroid hormone surges (or a transient hyperthyroidism known as thyrotoxicosis or Hashitoxicosis), as well as mood alterations, followed by an onset of hypothyroidism.

Hypothyroidism, in turn, is connected with brain fog, depression, fatigue, low libido, and pain.

Additionally, even when thyroid hormones are normal, as both Graves' and Hashimoto's are autoimmune inflammatory conditions, thyroid antibodies and inflammation can lead to numerous symptoms.

It is not uncommon for my thyroid clients to report feeling moody, depressed, anxious, and irritable when their thyroid hormone levels and thyroid antibodies are out of balance.

Doctors don't always do a full thyroid panel and don't always interpret thyroid labs correctly.

I have included a list of tests that constitute the full thyroid panel, as well as optimal reference ranges in the chart below.

Test	Standard Reference Range	Optimal Reference Range
TSH	0.4–5.5 µIU/mL	0.5–2 µIU/mL 0.5–2.5 µIU/mL in elderly
Free T4	9–23 pmol/L	15–23 pmol/L
Free T3	3–7 pmol/L	5–7 pmol/L
Reverse T3	11–21 ng/dL	11–18 ng/dL
TPO Antibodies	<35 IU/ml	<2 IU/ml
TG Antibodies	<35 IU/ml	<2 IU/ml

Understanding your labs

TSH. If your TSH is elevated, this may mean you need to talk to your doctor about starting or increasing thyroid hormones.

If your TSH is low, and you take thyroid medications, your doctor may need to lower your dose.

If your TSH is under 0.4 µIU/mL and/or you have symptoms of hyperthyroidism (and don't take any thyroid medications), you may also want to test for Graves' antibodies: TSI antibodies (sometimes called TSH receptor antibodies) and TBII *(thyrotropin binding inhibiting immunoglobulins).*

T3 and reverse T3. Inadequate or excess amounts of the active thyroid hormone T3 may also lead to issues with mood, fatigue, brain fog, and pain.

If your T3 is too low, or reverse T3 is too high, you may want to talk to your doctor about switching thyroid medications (or adjusting the dose).

The most commonly prescribed thyroid medications contain only T4, a pro-hormone that is converted to T3 in the body. Unfortunately, for a variety of reasons, some genetic, some individuals do not convert T4 to T3 properly. Fortunately, medication options that contain T3 are available. Some people find a resolution of lifelong depression simply by adding a T3-containing medication to their regimen.

High T3 can cause pain, including carpal tunnel syndrome, and may mean you need to lower your dose of thyroid medication.

Elevated thyroid antibodies. Supplementing with selenium can help reduce antibodies and can be a helpful tool for anxiety and OCD. One study found that over the course of three months, thyroid antibodies can be reduced by 40 percent. Many of my clients report feeling a new sense of calm.

Another small study in 2013 and a follow-up study in 2017 showed that thyroid antibodies and an elevated TSH could be significantly improved by using a combination of selenium and myo-inositol.

If you are taking the ATP supplements, you can switch up your myo-inositol for the Rootcology supplement that contains selenium and myo-inositol, Rootcology Selenium + Myo-Inositol, or simply add the Pure Encapsulations Selenium (selenomethionine) at 200–400 mcg per day to the Myo-Inositol that is a part of the program.

I have a website dedicated to helping people optimize their hormones and get into remission from Hashimoto's hypothyroidism—www.thyroid pharmacist.com—and wrote an entire eBook on how to optimize thyroid hormones, titled *Optimizing Thyroid Hormones*.

You can download the *Optimizing Thyroid Hormones* eBook for free on my website at http://thyroidpharmacist.com/atpbookbonus.

Please see my three books on Hashimoto's for detailed guidance on the root cause of Hashimoto's, protocols, and more Paleo recipes so that you can take charge of your thyroid health.

Hashimoto's Thyroiditis: Lifestyle Interventions for Finding and Treating the Root Cause by Izabella Wentz

Hashimoto's Protocol: A 90-Day Plan for Reversing Thyroid Symptoms and Getting Your Life Back by Izabella Wentz

Hashimoto's Food Pharmacology: Nutrition Protocols and Healing Recipes to Take Charge of Your Thyroid Health by Izabella Wentz

NUTRIENT GUIDE
Copper Toxicity
Related Stress Symptoms:
- Brain fog and fatigue (BFF)
- Insomnia and sleep issues (ISI)
- Mood (M)

Our bodies need a certain amount of copper to be healthy. Too little copper is harmful and can occur due to our not taking in enough copper or not absorbing it well. On the other hand, too much copper is also harmful, which can occur by taking in too much or not detoxing it well.

Most of the copper our body takes in comes from the foods we eat. High-copper foods include shellfish, oysters, nuts, seeds, and chocolate. We can also absorb copper from our water (that we drink or even bathe in) and metal pipes and products (copper cookware). Certain medications (oral contraceptives, antacids, copper-rich multivitamins), excess estrogen (due to natural hormone levels, estrogen dominance, or exposure to man-made estrogens found in meats, plastics, and personal care products), copper IUDs, and zinc deficiency can increase our exposure.

If someone is taking in too much copper or is not detoxing it well (due to gallbladder and liver impairment or other issues such as adrenal insufficiency or zinc deficiency), copper toxicity can occur. Many people with adrenal dysfunction have a congested liver, so that is likely one reason copper toxicity is a common root cause.

Common symptoms of copper toxicity include:

- Anxiety
- Fatigue
- Irritability, depression, tantrums
- Emotional lability, prone to rapid changes in emotional highs and lows, with exaggerated changes in mood (laughing one minute, crying or having a temper tantrum the next)
- Having a racing mind
- Insomnia (even with extreme fatigue)
- Hair turning orange or having a reddish tint
- Acne
- Poor concentration
- Skin rashes
- Poor wound healing
- Frequent colds/flu
- PMS symptoms
- White spots on fingernails

- Craving high-copper foods (such as chocolate)
- Dark blotches on face, especially during pregnancy (when estrogen levels are high)

Testing

There are a few options to test. The zinc and copper serum tests are usually the most accessible, as long as one knows how to interpret the results.

Blood tests:
- CMP-low alkaline phosphatase can indicate a potential zinc deficiency
- Zinc, plasma or serum
- Copper, serum

Test	Reference range	Ideal range
Zinc, plasma or serum	56–134 µg/dl	120–130 µg/dl
Copper, serum	72–166 µg/dl	70–120 µg/dl

Urine test:

Genova Diagnostics Comprehensive Urine Element Profile provoked with DMPS/DMSA to test for elevations in copper.

Hair test (tissue mineral analysis):

Elevated copper may show up directly or be hidden, where copper looks normal but results show high calcium and low zinc-to-copper ratio (less than 6:1), or high calcium and high mercury.

Dietary Recommendations

In general, you'll want to eat a diet that avoids high-copper foods and includes high-zinc foods. Zinc reduces the amount of copper your body absorbs and uses.

- High-copper foods (AVOID): organ meats like liver, oysters, spirulina, shiitake mushrooms, nuts and seeds, tofu, sweet potatoes, lobster, leafy greens, chocolate, avocados, beer, black tea, coffee.

- Foods that deplete zinc (AVOID): dairy, wheat, grains, dried fruit, beer, alcohol.
- High-zinc foods: nonorgan meats, eggs, poultry.

Supplement Recommendations
As always, please work with your local practitioner to determine the appropriate supplements and dosages for your individual needs. Recommended supplements (in order of priority):

Copper-free multivitamin: Pure Encapsulations Nutrient 950, copper-, iodine-, and iron-free version, six per day.

Zinc picolinate: Pure Encapsulations, 30–60 mg per day to displace copper.

Molybdenum: Douglas Laboratories, 100–500 mcg per day to clear copper from the bloodstream.

Manganese: Pure Encapsulations, 5–15 mg per day to displace copper from the liver.

Ferritin/Iron: Test and supplement if deficient as per page 359. Iron can displace copper from the liver.

Vitamin C: NOW Foods Chewable C-500, 500–3,000 mg per day to chelate copper.

B$_6$ (Pyridoxine): Douglas Laboratories, 50–200 mg per day or Rootcology P$_5$P (activated B$_6$), 50–200 mg to aid with symptoms of copper toxicity.

Alpha-lipoic acid: Pure Encapsulations, 50–150 mg per day to chelate copper.

Evening primrose oil: Pure Encapsulations, 500 mg twice per day to improve zinc absorption.

Magnesium citrate: Rootcology Magnesium Citrate Powder, Designs for Health MagCitrate Powder, or Pure Encapsulations Magnesium Citrate Capsules, 400 mg per day to help with anxiety associated with copper toxicity.

Please see *Why Am I So Tired?* by Ann Louise Gittleman for more guidance on copper toxicity.

Iron Toxicity/Overload
Related Stress Symptoms:
- Brain fog and fatigue (BFF)
- Insomnia and sleep issues (ISI)
- Libido (L)
- Mood (M)
- Pain (P)

Ferritin above 200 ng/mL in women (300 ng/mL in men) can be an indication of iron toxicity/iron overload.

- Symptoms include extreme fatigue, weakness, heart flutters or irregular heartbeat, joint and stomach pain, irritability, depression.
- More common in men, postmenopausal women, people with genes for hemochromatosis types 1, 2, 3, 4, and people living at elevations above 5,000 feet.
- Can also be an indication of inflammation. Resolving the source of inflammation can help.
- Lifelong, therapeutic phlebotomies every few months to lower ferritin levels to optimal amounts are the standard of care.
- Moving to sea level can be curative within three to six months of moving for elevation-induced cases.
- IP6 (inositol hexaphosphate) supplement (Pure Encapsulations) may lower ferritin and reduce the need for therapeutic phlebotomies (may need to supplement calcium and zinc, as IP6 can lower them, too). Doses may vary.
- Milk thistle can help protect the liver from damage caused by excess iron (Pure Encapsulations Silymarin [milk thistle extract], 250 mg, one to four times per day).

- Lowering intake of dietary iron and eating phytates and oxalates with iron-rich foods may be helpful for some, but it is not usually curative and can also prevent the absorption of other nutrients such as zinc and calcium.

Nutrients

Signs and Symptoms of Nutrient Deficiency

Nutrient	Adrenal Symptom	Symptoms
Vitamin A	L	Dry, itchy skin, night blindness, fertility issues, frequent infections
B$_1$ (Thiamine)	BFF, P	Fatigue, low blood pressure, adrenal issues
B$_2$ (Riboflavin)	BFF, P, ISI	Cracks at the corners of the mouth, cracked lips, inflammation of the tongue and lining of the mouth, mouth ulcers, fatigue, migraines, anxiety, iron-deficiency anemia
B$_6$/P$_5$P	M, L, P	Skin rashes, cracked and sore lips, inflamed tongue, anxiety, depression, irritability, fatigue, pain in hands and feet
B$_{12}$	BFF, ISI, M	Fatigue, depression, neurological issues, brain fog, tingling extremities, nerve damage, digestive deficiencies, seizures, anemia
Vitamin C	BFF, ISI	Poor immune function, poor detoxification
Copper	BFF	Fatigue, weakness, frequent sickness, poor memory
Vitamin D	BFF	Low levels on test, autoimmunity, fatigue, bone aches, frequent illness or infections, muscle pain and weakness, depression
Ferritin/Iron	BFF, ISI, M	Low levels on test, hair loss, breathlessness, fatigue, anemia, mood swings

Nutrient	Adrenal Symptom	Symptoms
Folate (Vitamin B$_9$)	BFF, ISI, M	Elevated homocysteine, birth defects, tongue grooves, anemia, brain fog, depression, fatigue, insomnia, low energy, muscle weakness, heavy menses, multiple miscarriages, bright red rash under nose
Magnesium	BFF, P, ISI	Headaches, constipation, pain, insomnia, muscle cramps, anxiety, reflux
Omega-3	M, BFF, P	Dry skin, eczema, mood, dandruff, stiffness
Selenium	M, BFF	Anxiety, hair loss, elevated thyroid antibodies
Zinc	M	Weight loss, brain fog, poor wound healing, diarrhea, loss of appetite

Nutrients That Require Testing

Many nutrients can be taken based on assessments of symptoms and do not require lab testing, due to their great safety record.

I recommend working with a practitioner to evaluate your need for the fat-soluble vitamins A, D, E, and K; copper; and ferritin, as these can build up to toxic levels. B$_{12}$ levels are important to test, as they can provide a signal for root causes that need to be addressed (pernicious anemia, diet, SIBO, H. pylori) and to ensure that oral absorption is occurring properly.

Tests for vitamins A, E, and K are not done routinely, but blood tests for B$_{12}$, copper, ferritin, and vitamin D can be ordered by your physician and covered by insurance. While it's not required to test homocysteine or for the MTHFR (methylenetetrahydrofolate reductase) gene before supplementing with folate (as methylfolate, the most bioavailable version), these tests may help with determining dosage and the need for additional interventions.

If you don't have a doctor who can order the labs for you, you can self-order each of the labs separately, or you can order the full Root Cause Nutrition panel from Ulta Lab Tests.

Nutrient	Test	Recommended Products, Dose, and Notes
B$_{12}$	Vitamin B$_{12}$ (Cobalamin) Standard reference range: 200–900 pg/mL Optimal reference range: 700–800 pg/mL	Pure Encapsulations B$_{12}$ sublingual, 5,000 mcg under the tongue daily for ten days, then 5,000 mcg under the tongue once per week for four weeks, then 5,000 mcg under the tongue monthly for maintenance (If you have the COMT V158M gene mutation or mitochondrial issues, the Adenosyl/Hydroxy B$_{12}$ liquid from Pure Encapsulations may work better.)
Iron	Ferritin (iron storage protein) Standard reference range: 12–150 ng/mL Optimal reference range: 90–110 ng/mL	For low ferritin: Thorne Research, Iron Bisglycinate, Designs for Health Ferrochel—Chelated Ferrous Iron, Pure Encapsulations OptiFerin-C. Follow package instructions or your practitioner's advice. Iron supplements are the most common supplements indicated in overdose.
Vitamin D	25-Hydroxyvitamin D Standard reference range: 30–100 ng/mL Optimal reference range: 60–80 ng/mL	Pure Encapsulations Vitamin D, 5,000–10,000 IU per day, retest within three to six months of starting

Nutrients That Do Not Require Lab Testing

Supplement	Symptoms	Recommended Product, Dose, and Notes
B-complex	BFF, M, P	Pure Encapsulations B-Complex Plus, one per day
Choline	BFF, ISI	Vital Nutrients Citicoline, 500–2,000 mg daily
Chromium	ISI	Pure Encapsulations ChromeMate GTF, 600 mcg per day
Coenzyme Q$_{10}$	BFF, P	Pure Encapsulations CoQ$_{10}$, 200–500 mg per day
D-ribose	BFF, P	Pure Encapsulations Ribose, 250 mg–15 grams per day
Evening primrose oil	M, L	Pure Encapsulations E.P.O. (evening primrose oil), 500 mg twice per day

Supplement	Symptoms	Recommended Product, Dose, and Notes
Fulvic acid	BFF	Jarrow Shilajit Fulvic Acid Complex, one capsule, one or two times per day with a meal
Glycine	BFF, ISI	Designs for Health Glycine Powder, 3 grams per day
Manganese	BFF	Pure Encapsulations Manganese, 5–15 mg per day
Methylfolate with cofactors	M	Rootcology MTHFR Pathways, one or two per day Pure Encapsulations Homocysteine Factors, one or two per day Designs for Health Homocysteine Supreme, one or two per day
Molybdenum	M	Douglas Laboratories Molybdenum, 100–500 mcg per day
N-acetyl-cysteine (NAC)	BFF, L, M, P	Rootcology Pure N-Acetyl Cysteine, Pure Encapsulations NAC, Designs for Health N-Acetyl-Cysteine, 1,800 mg daily with food
Nutritional lithium	M	Pure Encapsulations Lithium (orotate). Recommended doses range from 400 mcg to 10 mg. (Work with your medical practitioner to determine the proper dose.) While pharmaceutical lithium can be toxic to the thyroid gland, nutritional lithium seems to be better tolerated. That said, be sure to check thyroid function after starting.
Omega-3 fatty acids	BFF, M, P	Pure Encapsulations EPA/DHA Essentials or Designs for Health OmegAvai Synergy, 1–4 grams per day Nordic Naturals Arctic Cod Liver Oil, 1 teaspoon daily

Supplement	Symptoms	Recommended Product, Dose, and Notes
Selenium	BFF, M	Rootcology Selenium + Myo-Inositol, one capsule per day Pure Encapsulations Selenium (selenomethionine), 200–400 mcg per day Selenium is a nutrient with a narrow therapeutic index, so the dose has to be just right to ensure efficacy and prevent toxicity. Doses of 200–400 mcg per day are considered safe and beneficial for most people, while those above 800 mcg are considered toxic.
Thiamine (vitamin B$_1$)	BFF, ISI, P	Pure Encapsulations BenfoMax, 600 mg per day You may need to increase your dosage of thiamine if your weight is above 60 kilograms (132 pounds). While 600 mg is a good daily starting dosage, one study on the effect of thiamine on patients with Crohn's disease and ulcerative colitis published in the *Journal of Alternative and Complementary Medicine* found that effective dosages ranged from 600 to 1,500 mg per day, depending on the body size of the individuals. Higher doses may be associated with reversible dose-related adverse reactions, including a rapid heartbeat (tachycardia). I encourage you to work with a practitioner to determine the proper dosage for your needs.
Trimethylglycine (TMG)	BFF, P	Allergy Research Group TMG, 2.5 grams per day
Vitamin B$_6$	BFF, ISI, L, M, P	Pyridoxine: Douglas Laboratories B$_6$ P$_5$P (the active form): Rootcology P$_5$P Designs for Health P-5-P Pure Encapsulations P$_5$P 50 Klaire Labs Vitamin B$_6$ 50–200 mg/day. Do not use more than 300 mg/day of B$_6$ in the pyridoxine form.

Supplement	Symptoms	Recommended Product, Dose, and Notes
Vitamin C	BFF, L, M	NOW Foods C-500 Chewable tablets (cherry or orange flavor), 500–3,000 mg per day
Vitamin E	BFF	Integrative Therapeutics Vitamin E or NOW Sun-E 400, one per day
Zinc	L, M	Pure Encapsulations Zinc Picolinate, 30 mg per day (larger doses require a doctor's supervision)

Pyroluria

Related Stress Symptoms:

- Brain fog and fatigue (BFF)
- Insomnia and sleep issues (ISI)
- Mood (M)

Pyroluria is a lifestyle-induced abnormality in the synthesis of hemoglobin, the protein that binds iron in red blood cells, resulting in the production of too much hydroxyhemopyrrolin-2-one (HPL), also known as "pyrroles." The current scientific literature shows that pyrroles bind to zinc and vitamin B_6, causing them to be excreted through urine in large amounts and necessitating supplementation.

Pyroluria can cause:

- Shyness
- Introversion
- Social anxiety
- Fatigue
- Depression
- Cold hands or feet
- Reduced amount of hair on the head or prematurely gray hair
- Morning constipation
- Morning nausea or lack of appetite
- Poor dream recall

- Strange dreams or nightmares
- Depression
- Puffy, swollen face
- Iron anemia or having low ferritin

Urine tests can be helpful. However, pyroluria expert Trudy Scott shares that testing can come up with false negatives, so she always relies on assessments and response to supplements.

Dietary Recommendations

In general, you'll want to eat a diet that avoids high-copper foods (because zinc levels are often so low in people with pyroluria, copper levels become elevated) and foods that deplete zinc and vitamin B_6. Include foods high in arachidonic acid, an essential omega-6 fatty acid. Many people with pyroluria are low in omega-6s.

- Avoid high-copper foods, including organ meats like liver, oysters, spirulina, shiitake mushrooms, nuts and seeds, tofu, sweet potatoes, lobster, leafy greens, chocolate, avocados, beer, black tea, coffee.
- Avoid foods that deplete zinc and vitamin B_6, including dairy, wheat, grains, dried fruit, beer, alcohol.

Supplement Recommendations

Start with:

- Zinc picolinate: Pure Encapsulations, 30 mg at breakfast (with food).
- B_6 (Pyridoxine): Douglas Laboratories B_6, 100 mg; or Rootcology P_5P, 50 mg (activated B_6).
- Evening primrose oil: Pure Encapsulations E.P.O., 1,300 mg, to aid the absorption of zinc.

Every week for the next four weeks, evaluate your body's response. If you are feeling great on the starting dose and your social anxiety is gone, you should stay at that dose.

- If your zinc levels are not going up (based on the liquid zinc sulfate test), increase to 60 mg.
- Evaluate dream recall each week and, if needed, increase B_6 by 100 mg each week up to 500 mg. You should aim for having pleasant dreams where you wake up and want to return to them, and remember them later in the day.
- If there is no improvement in how you feel and in dream recall once you reach 300 mg B_6, then switch to P_5P (pyridoxal-5-phosphate), the active form of B_6.

Please see *The Antianxiety Food Solution* by Trudy Scott for more information.

PROBIOTICS
Related Stress Symptoms:
- Brain fog and fatigue (BFF)
- Insomnia and sleep issues (ISI)
- Mood (M)

A supplement of the beneficial yeast *Saccharomyces boulardii* is recommended as part of the ATP. These are other types of probiotics that may also be helpful.

Lactobacillus-Based High-Dose Multi-Strain Probiotics
I recommend taking a multi-strain probiotic with various strains of *Lactobacillus, Bifidobacteria,* and in some cases, beneficial *Streptococcus* bacteria instead of single-strain probiotics that contain only one type of *Lactobacillus*.

- Avoid high-dose multi-strain probiotics if you have SIBO, which can be caused by an overgrowth of various bacteria, including *Lactobacillus* and *Streptococcus* bacteria.
- If you have obsessive thoughts, avoid probiotics that contain *Streptococcus* probiotic strains—they can theoretically increase obsessive-compulsive symptoms.

- It's important to note that drugstore probiotics often have doses too low for making health shifts, so higher doses may be needed, but one may need to start low and go slow.
- If you've never taken probiotics, you will want to start with a 10 billion CFU probiotic and work your way up to a higher dose, like 50 billion CFU, over time.
  - Rootcology ProB 50
  - Pure Encapsulations 50B
  - Designs for Health ProbioMed 50

Soil-Based Probiotics

Soil-based probiotics are naturally occurring, spore-based, and have a unique mechanism of action, which allows them to directly modulate the gut microbiome.

- Spore-based probiotics have shown promise in various autoimmune diseases, as well as in reducing allergies and asthma.
- They also have an ability to boost *Lactobacillus* colonies, so they can be used concurrently with *Lactobacillus* probiotics, as well as in place of them.
- Unlike the *Lactobacillus* probiotics, spore-based probiotics can reduce SIBO and increase gut diversity by boosting the growth of other beneficial flora.
- Options include:
  - Rootcology Spore Flora: A unique formulation with five different bacillus strains that can produce enzymes, secretory proteins, antimicrobial compounds, vitamins, and carotenoids that are able to withstand stomach acid's low pH, allowing for improved delivery. The starting dose is half a capsule per day, then increase to one full capsule after one week.
  - Microbiome Labs MegaSporeBiotic: The starting dose is one capsule every other day, and the therapeutic dose is two capsules per day. Once the desired effect has been seen, practitioners recommend dropping down to a maintenance dose of one capsule per day.

Remember, always start low and go slow with probiotics. You may have increased symptoms if your gut flora changes too rapidly.

SELECTED HERBS

Supplement	Symptoms	Recommended Product, Dose, and Notes
Chaste Tree (Vitex)	ISI, L	Pure Encapsulations Chaste Tree (Vitex), one capsule, twice daily
Lion's Mane	BFF	Four Sigmatic Lion's Mane Mushroom Elixir, one packet a day
Maca	BFF, L	Femmenessence, follow package instructions
Rhodiola	BFF	Pure Encapsulations Rhodiola Rosea, 100 mg, one or two times per day
Shatavari	BFF, L	Organic India Shatavari, one or two capsules, two times per day
Turmeric	L, M, P	Rootcology Curcumin Absorb, one capsule per day Designs for Health Curcum-Evail, one capsule per day Pure Encapsulations Curcumin 500 with Bioperine, one capsule, one to three times daily

How to Modify the Program

FOOD SENSITIVITY SUBSTITUTION GUIDE

If you have known sensitivities to any of the foods recommended on the ATP diet, here's a list of potential substitutions:

Common Ingredients That May Pose a Sensitivity	Approved Ingredient Substitutions
Avocado	Chia seeds, coconut oil, extra-virgin olive oil
Chia seeds	Gelatin, avocado (smoothies)
Coconut flour (for thickening)	Arrowroot flour, tapioca flour
Coconut milk	Nut and seed milk (additive-free)
Coconut oil	Avocado oil, extra-virgin olive oil, grass-fed animal lard, palm-oil shortening (sustainable)
Eggs	Hydrolyzed beef protein, pea protein, flaxseeds, chia seeds
Fermented coconut water	Coconut water, sparkling water
Lemon	Lime or 1 teaspoon apple cider vinegar (in 1 cup of water)
Nut milks	Coconut milk
Orange juice in Adrenal Kick Start (page 297) (alternative high vitamin C options)	½ cup of tart cherry juice, ½ cup of acerola cherry juice (may be difficult to source), ⅓ cup of organic strawberries (blended with ¼ cup of water), 1 organic kiwi (blended with ¼ cup of water). See page 297 for the full recipe.
Stevia	Honey, maple syrup, monk fruit (small amounts)

FOOD SENSITIVITY TESTING

To test for your unique food sensitivities, I've found the Alletess Lab 96 Comprehensive Food Panel and Alletess Lab 184 Comprehensive Food Panel to be highly accurate.

SLOW SUPPLEMENT INTRODUCTION GUIDE FOR SENSITIVE INDIVIDUALS

If you tend to be sensitive to supplements, I recommend introducing one supplement at a time, every three to seven days, to make sure you are tolerating them. You will start with the first supplement, at the lowest dose, and slowly increase your dosage, day by day, until you reach the target dose or the dose you can comfortably tolerate. You will want to be at the full dose or at your target dose for three full days before continuing on to the next supplement. This is why it can take up to seven days before a new supplement is introduced.

ATP Diet-Compliant Protein Powder

- Start with a half serving, for three days.
- If you don't feel well, remove it from your regimen and find an alternate protein that you tolerate. For guidelines, refer to Choosing a Protein Powder (page 113).
- If you feel well, increase to one serving the following day.
- If you don't feel well, decrease back to half a serving the following day.

Electrolyte Blend

- Start with half a scoop, for three days.
- If you don't feel well, remove it from your regimen.
- If you feel well, increase to one scoop the following day.
- If you don't feel well, decrease back to the half-scoop dose the following day.

Magnesium Citrate

If taking a powder:

- Start with ¼ teaspoon at bedtime, for three days.
- If you don't feel well, remove it from your regimen.

- If you feel well, increase to ½ teaspoon the following day.
- If you feel well, increase to 1 teaspoon the following day.
- If you don't feel well, decrease to ½ teaspoon the following day.

If taking capsules:
- Start with one capsule at bedtime, for three days.
- If you don't feel well, remove it from your regimen.
- If you feel well, increase to two capsules the following day.
- If you don't feel well, decrease back to one capsule the following day.

Carnitine Blend
- Start with one capsule with breakfast, for three days.
- If you don't feel well, remove it from your regimen.
- If you feel well, add one capsule with dinner the following day.
- If you feel well, take two capsules with breakfast and one with dinner the following day.
- If you feel well, take two capsules with breakfast and two with dinner the following day.
- If you don't feel well, decrease to the last dose you felt well with on the following day.

Adrenal Support Supplement
- Start with one capsule at breakfast, for three days.
- If you don't feel well, remove it from your regimen and return to Supplement Spotlight #1: Adrenal Support Blend (page 118) for guidance on alternative blends that may work better for you.
- If you feel well, take two capsules at breakfast the following day.
- If you feel well, take three capsules at breakfast the following day.
- If you don't feel well, decrease to the last dose you felt well with on the following day.

Myo-Inositol
- Start with ⅛ teaspoon at dinner, for three days.
- If you don't feel well, remove it from your regimen.
- If you feel well, take ¼ teaspoon at dinner the following day.

- If you don't feel well, decrease back to ⅛ teaspoon at dinner the following day.

Saccharomyces boulardii
- Start with ½ capsule at breakfast, for three days.
- If you don't feel well, remove it from your regimen.
- If you feel well, increase to one capsule at breakfast the following day.
- If you feel well, add one capsule with dinner the following day.
- If you don't feel well, decrease to the last dose you felt well with on the following day.

Signs of a Reaction
Generally, any changes with supplements should be positive. You may experience some slightly uncomfortable symptoms as your body adjusts, but they should be tolerable and subside within a few days. Please listen to your body. If they don't ease up, discontinue using the supplements.

If you experience any of the following adverse reactions, please discontinue the supplement(s) immediately and follow up with your practitioner:

Vomiting

Rash or itching

Bleeding, nose bleeds

Shortness of breath, wheezing

Sudden/severe headaches

Sudden/severe swelling

Testing

Testing For	Recommended Tests
Addison's disease	· Sodium, potassium, cortisol levels, ACTH stimulation tests, 21-hydroxylase antibodies (adrenal antibodies) · Imaging of the adrenals
Adrenal dysfunction	· Precision Analytical DUTCH (Dried Urine Test for Comprehensive Hormones) Plus · ZRT Laboratory Adrenal Stress Test Kit
Comprehensive stool analysis that tests for dysbiosis, pathogenic bacteria like *H. pylori* and strep, and parasites like *Blastocystis hominis*	· Diagnostic Solutions GI-MAP · Great Plains Laboratory Comprehensive Stool Analysis · Doctor's Data Comprehensive Stool Analysis · Genova Diagnostics GI Effects Comprehensive Profile—Stool · Vibrant Wellness Gut Zoomer 3.0
Copper toxicity	· Copper, serum · Zinc, plasma or serum
Epstein-Barr Reactivation	· EBV Early Antigen
Female hormones	· Blood tests: progesterone (test on day 21 of cycle in menstruating women), testosterone, and estradiol · Precision Analytical DUTCH (Dried Urine Test for Comprehensive Hormones) Complete
Food sensitivity tests found to be highly accurate for myself and my clients	· Alletess Lab 96 Comprehensive Food Panel or · Alletess Lab 184 Comprehensive Food Panel

Testing For	Recommended Tests

Foundational Nutrient Panel	· CBC (Complete Blood Count)
	   Please note, low alkaline phosphatase on
	   a CBC may indicate low zinc
	
	   · CMP (Comprehensive Metabolic Panel)
	   · Ferritin
	   · Homocysteine
	   · Vitamin B_{12}
	   · Vitamin D, 1,25-Dihydroxy

Mold	· For body colonization
	   · Great Plains Laboratory Organic Acids
	   Test
	   · Great Plains Laboratory MycoTOX Profile
	· Home testing
	   · ImmunoLytics
	   · ERMI

Organic acids tests can reveal yeast, mold, *Candida* and *Clostridia* metabolites, elevated ammonia, neurotransmitter metabolites, deficiencies in riboflavin, mitochondrial issues, and many other root causes	Great Plains Laboratory Organic Acids Test
SIBO	Breath tests (Commonwealth Laboratories and Genova Diagnostics)
Toxicity	· GPL-TOX Profile · Great Plains Laboratory Glyphosate Test · Great Plains Laboratory Metals Hair Test

You can order most of these labs through your practitioner. If you are looking for self-order options, I have set up a few links for you:

Blood Tests: Ulta Labs—ultalabtests.com/thyroidpharmacist

Functional Medicine Test Kits (including the GI-MAP test for gut infections): Rupa Health—rupahealth.com/practitioner-catalogs/hashimotos-self-management-program and DirectLabs—directlabs.com/thyroidrx

Alletess Food Sensitivity Tests: MyMedLab—thyroidrx.mymedlab.com

Index

Note: *Italicized* page numbers indicate material in tables or illustrations.